Illustrated Review of
NEUROANATOMY

3 Dimensional Perspective

Josephine Anthony, Ph.D
Simon Fraser University
Burnaby, B.C.

Illustrations and cover design: Paul DeGrace
Desktop Publishing: Monica Hartanto
Photography: Malcolm Toms

6th Edition

ISBN 9781077336001

Simon Fraser University

Simon Fraser University
Burnaby, B.C.

PREFACE

"An Illustrated Review of Neuroanatomy, a 3 Dimensional perspective" is written from the perspective of a student. It is designed to help the student learn the material, comprehend the subject, develop concepts and reinforce the understanding of neuroanatomical entities from a functional viewpoint. Review of each topic will help the student correlate information for understanding of basic concepts. Text-Illustration combination will be effective in visualization and orientation of structures. There is also the option of applying contrasting colors to aid distinction between distinct anatomical entities. This will help the student to distinguish structures and pathways in each region, reduce complexity of structures, facilitate learning, as well as providing an opportunity for self evaluation. All students will benefit equally, finding it easier to understand the 3D perspective and be challenged to supplement learning with group discussions.. It would also help students to observe details that otherwise would not have been obvious, allowing a visual journey through various areas of the brain.

The strengths of this manual are:

- 3D labeled diagrams of structures and pathways that are sequential in nature
- Covers all regions of the brain from a functional and anatomical viewpoint
- Easily understandable, since structures shown in its entirety from origin to termination
- Outline of various topics and appropriate diagrams accompanying each description
- Various structures and pathways can be color-coded for ease of identification
- Easy review of each topic and therefore would complement any neuroanatomy text.
- Pathways and structures can be identified and located accurately in dissections of the brain.
- Illustrations depicted in this manual are drawn as it appears *in situ*

ACKNOWLEDGMENTS

I am indebted to Paul DeGrace for his painstaking work in rendering a superb reproduction of simple neuroanatomy drawings. The computerized versions of these drawings attests to Paul's delicate handiwork, allowing an appreciation of structures in the 3 dimension. I acknowledge with deep appreciation Paul's perseverance and his dedication to perfection.

I gratefully acknowledge Vicky Earle's artistic interpretation of neuroanatomy and for editing all diagrams, placing complex structures in 3-dimensional planes

I am particularly grateful to Bill Schuss for helping to initiate this endeavor, he was challenged to apply his artistic skills to produce computerized drawings of complex neuroanatomical structures.

Heartfelt thanks to Malcolm Toms for his help and expertise in capturing the essence of the brain in photographs included in this publication. I also wish to thank all who supported me on this project.

All of the illustrations were drawn by the author and the following texts were referenced:
Kiernan, JA: Barr's The Human Nervous System An Anatomical Viewpoint, 9th ed., Lippincott Williams & Wilkins, Philadelphia; 2009; Haines, DE: Neuroanatomy An Atlas of Structures, Sections and Systems, 7th ed., Lippincott Williams & Wilkins, Philadelphia; 2008; Siegel, A and Sapru, HN: Essential Neuroscience 1st ed., Lippincott Williams & Wilkins, Philadelphia; 2006; Martin, JH: Neuroanatomy Text and Atlas, 3rd ed., The McGraw-Hill Companies Inc. N.Y., 2003; Bhatnagar,SC: Neuroscience For the Study of Communicative Diseases, 2nd ed., Lippincott Williams & Wilkins, Philadelphia; 2002; Lockhart, RD, Hamilton, GF and Fyfe FW: Anatomy of the Human Body, 2nd ed., Faber & Faber Ltd., 1965; Afifi, AK and Bergman, RA: Functional Neuroanatomy Text and Atlas, 2nd ed., The McGraw-Hill Companies Inc. N.Y. 2005; Woolsey, TA, Hanaway,J, Gado,MH: The Brain Atlas A visual Guide to the Human Central Nervous System, 3rd ed., John Wiley & Sons, Inc., New Jersey, 2005; Steward, O: Functional Neuroscience, 1st ed., Springer-Verlag N.Y. 2000; Nolte,J: The Human Brain An Introduction to Its Functional Anatomy, 5th ed., Mosby, Inc N.Y. 2002; Agur, AMR: Grant's Atlas of Anatomy, 11th ed., Lippincott Williams & Wilkins, Philadelphia; 2005; Fix, HD: High-yield Neuroanatomy, 2nd ed., Lippincott Williams & Wilkins, Philadelphia; 2000; Pansky, B. Allen, DJ: Review of Neuroscience, 1st ed., Macmillan Publishing Co. Inc. N.Y.; Nieuwenhuys,R., Voogd,J, van Huijzen, C: The human central nervous system, A synopsis and Atlas, 2nd ed., Springer-Verlag, Berlin, 1981; Spalteholz, W; Spanner,R: Atlas of Human Anatomy, 16th ed., Scheltema & Holkema NV, Amsterdam, 1967; Netter, FH: The Ciba Collection of Medical Illustrations Volume 1, Nervous System, 5th ed., Ciba Pharmaceutical Company, Summit, NJ, 1962; Standring, S: Gray's Anatomy, 39th ed., Elsevier Churchill Livingstone, Edinburgh, 2005

TABLE OF CONTENTS

CHAPTER
1

DEVELOPMENT AND ORGANIZATION
OF THE NERVOUS SYSTEM

Overview

The nervous system develops during the third week of development, as a longitudinal tube, the **neural tube**. The neural tube gives rise to the central nervous system and its cavity forms the ventricular system of the brain. Cells that migrate from the neural tube, the **neural crest cells** give rise to the peripheral nervous system.

The major divisions of the nervous system are the ***central nervous system*** and the ***peripheral nervous system***. The central nervous system includes the spinal cord, medulla oblongata, pons, midbrain, cerebellum, diencephalon and the cerebrum. The peripheral nervous system includes the cranial and spinal nerves and the autonomic nervous system

The following account is restricted to the major events of the development of the nervous system.

I. Development of the Nervous System:

Following fertilization, the zygote undergoes a series of rapid succession of mitotic divisions to form a solid sphere of cells referred to as the **morula** (Figure 1.1). The morula gives rise to an ***inner cell mass*** and a ***blastocyst cavity.*** Following implantation, the inner cell mass differentiates into the ***endoderm*** and the ***ectoderm***, which together form the bilaminar embryonic disc. At the 3rd week of development, the bilaminar embryonic disc becomes a trilaminar embryonic disc consisting of three primary germ layers. These are the ***ectoderm***, ***mesoderm*** and ***endoderm*** (Figure 1.2). The primary germ layers give rise to various tissues and organs of the body.

A. Formation of the Neural plate:

1. Formation of the Brain:

- the dorsal ectoderm (**neurectoderm**), in the midline of the embryo, thickens to form the ***neural plate*** (Figure 1.3)
- lateral edges of the neural plate elevate inward to form the ***neural folds***. The midline groove between the neural folds is the ***neural groove***

- neural folds fuse to form the **neural tube.** The cranial part of the neural tube becomes the brain and the remaining part becomes the spinal cord
- the opening at the rostral end of the neural tube is the **anterior neuropore** and at the caudal end of the neural tube is the **posterior neuropore.** The anterior and posterior neuropores close at about the end of week four
- as the neural tube forms, some cells migrate from the lateral ridges of the neural plate to form the **neural crest.** Cells of the neural crest lie external to the neural tube.
- increased cell migration and unequal growth rates form flexures and three enlargements at the anterior end of the neural tube. The three primary divisions (Figure 1.4) of the brain are the **prosencephalon** (forebrain), **mesencephalon** (midbrain) and **rhombencephalon** (hindbrain).
- as development proceeds, secondary swellings appear in the prosencephalon and rhombencephalon.
- the *prosencephalon* forms:
    - the **telencephalon** and the **diencephalon**
    - the cavity develops into the **lateral ventricle** *and* **third ventricle** respectively
- the *mesencephalon* forms:
    - the **midbrain**.
    - the cavity develops into the **cerebral aqueduct**
- the·*rhombencephalon* forms:
    - the **metencephalon**, which develops into the **pons** and **cerebellum**
    - **myelencephalon**, which develops into the **medulla oblongata**
    - the cavity develops into the **fourth ventricle**

2. Formation of the Spinal cord:

- the lateral walls of the caudal part of the neural tube thicken by mitosis and proliferation of cells
- a longitudinal groove, the **sulcus limitans** appears in the lateral wall of the neural tube
- the sulcus limitans separates the **dorsal (alar) plates** from the **ventral (basal) plates,** these give rise to afferent and efferent connections, respectively (Figure 1.5)
- the dorsal or alar plate gives rise to the **dorsal gray horn** and the ventral or basal plate give rise to the **ventral gray horn.**

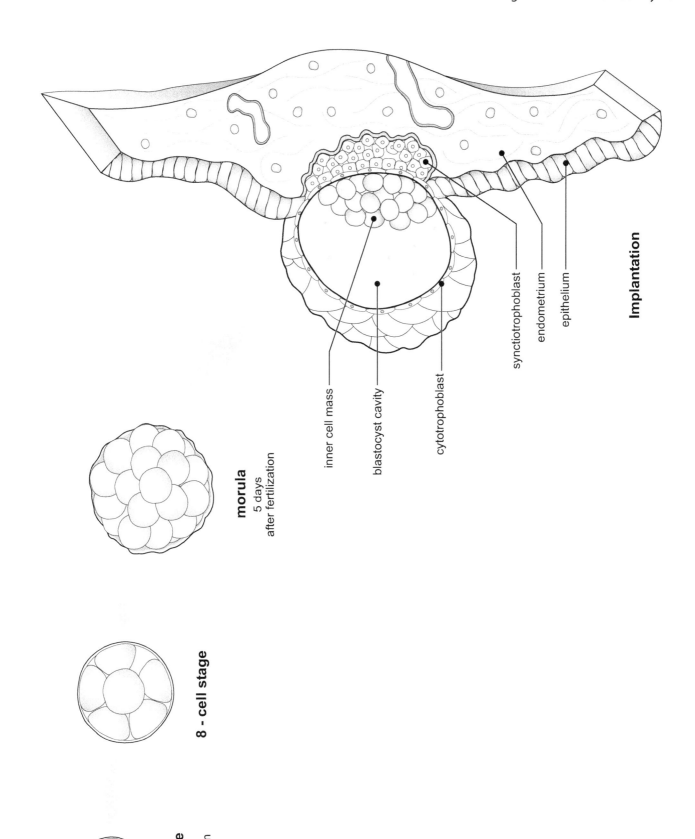

inner cell mass

blastocyst cavity

cytotrophoblast

synctiotrophoblast

endometrium

epithelium

Implantation

morula
5 days
after fertilization

8 - cell stage

2- cell stage
2-3 days
after fertilization

Figure 1.1 Formation of the morula and implantation in the endometrium

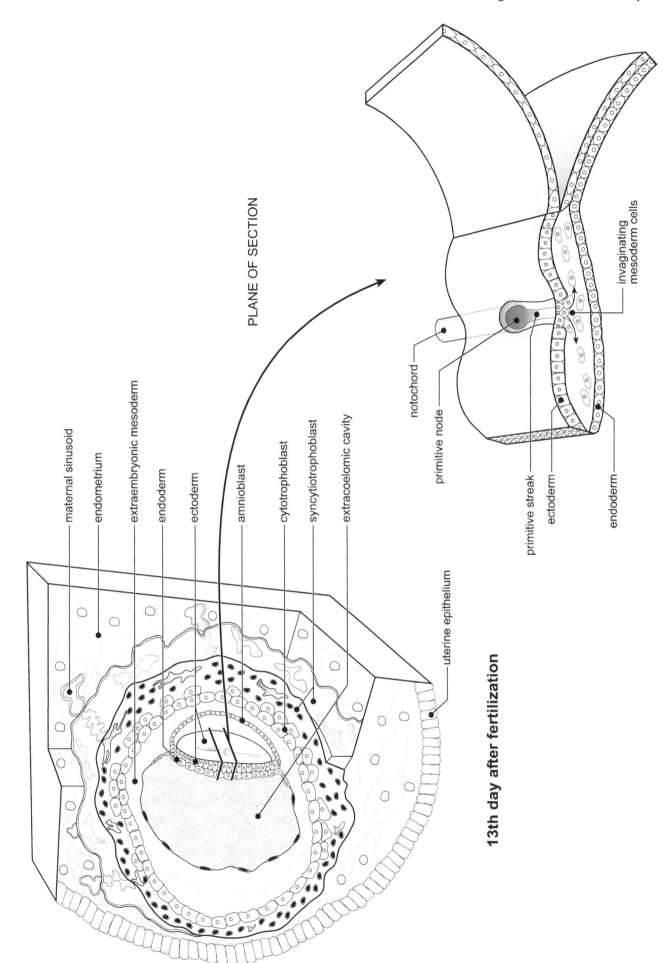

PLANE OF SECTION

maternal sinusoid

endometrium

extraembryonic mesoderm

endoderm

ectoderm

amnioblast

cytotrophoblast

syncytiotrophoblast

extracoelomic cavity

uterine epithelium

13th day after fertilization

notochord

primitive node

primitive streak

ectoderm

endoderm

invaginating
mesoderm cells

Figure 1.2   Formation of the trilaminar embryo

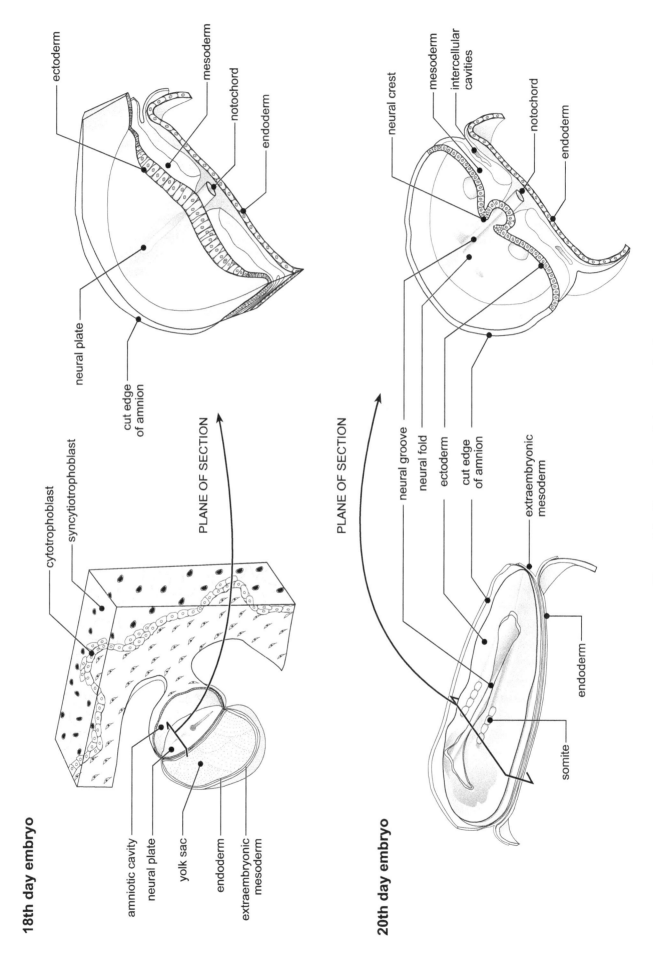

18th day embryo

20th day embryo

Figure 1.3 Formation of the neural tube

B. Neuronal Histogenesis:

    i. Cells of the neural tube form ***neuroblasts*** and ***glioblasts***
- neuroblasts give rise to almost all neurons of the central nervous system
- glioblasts give rise to astrocytes, oligodendrocytes and ependymal cells

    ii. the ***neural crest*** gives rise to the dorsal root ganglia; cranial nerve ganglia; autonomic ganglia and schwann cells

    iii. "functional" neurons once differentiated lose the capacity to undergo cell division; glial cells on the other hand, retain their ability to undergo cell division

    iv. development is influenced by neurochemical attractants (neurotransmitters, endorphins and nerve growth factors), interneuronal competition and synaptic formation.

    v. cell death occurs in the normal course of development. Between 40% and 75% of all neurons do not survive because they fail to make optimal synapses. Neuron death leads to synapse rearrangement

Clinical Notes:

Abnormal development of the Nervous System

    i. *anencephaly:*
- failure of closure of anterior neuropore
- absence of the forebrain, cranial vault and scalp

    ii. ***spina bifida occulta:***
- midline skeletal defect; vertebral laminae and vertebral arches fail to develop

    iii. ***hydrocephalus:***
- malformation of cerebral structures and obstruction of flow of cerebrospinal fluid
- results in increase skull size and increased intracranial pressure

II. General Organization of the Nervous System

Refer to Figure 1.6 for the major regions of the brain

A. Central Nervous System:

1. Spinal cord:

- consists of white matter that contain sensory tracts (ascending tracts) conveying sensory information from the periphery to areas of the brain. Motor tracts (descending tracts) convey impulses from the brain to neurons in the spinal gray matter
- consists of central core of gray matter that contains motor and sensory neurons and interneurons that play an important role in spinal reflexes
- impulses enter and leave the spinal cord through 31 pairs of spinal nerves that extend along the length of the cord

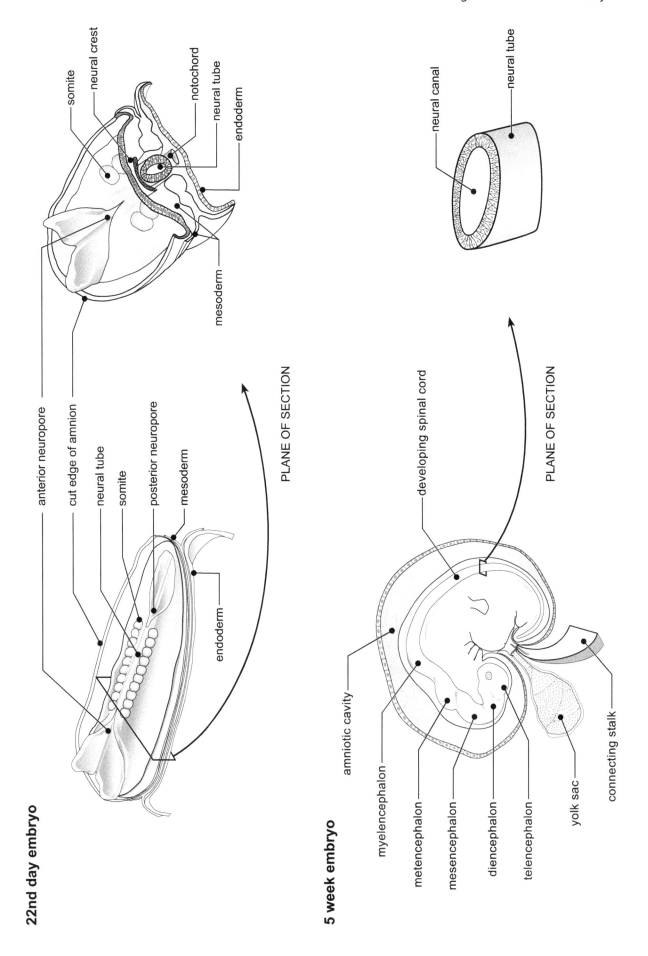

22nd day embryo

somite

neural crest

notochord

neural tube

endoderm

mesoderm

anterior neuropore

cut edge of amnion

neural tube

somite

posterior neuropore

mesoderm

endoderm

PLANE OF SECTION

5 week embryo

neural canal

neural tube

developing spinal cord

PLANE OF SECTION

amniotic cavity

myelencephalon

metencephalon

mesencephalon

diencephalon

telencephalon

yolk sac

connecting stalk

Figure 1.4   Development of the brain and spinal cord

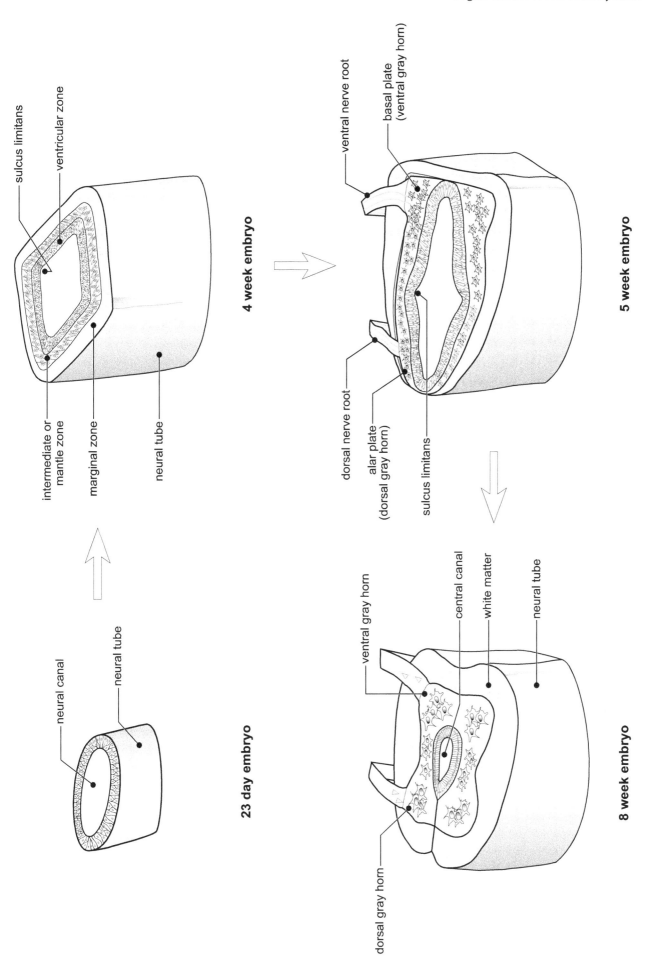

sulcus limitans

ventricular zone

intermediate or mantle zone

marginal zone

neural tube

4 week embryo

neural canal

neural tube

23 day embryo

ventral nerve root

basal plate (ventral gray horn)

dorsal nerve root

alar plate (dorsal gray horn)

sulcus limitans

5 week embryo

ventral gray horn

central canal

white matter

neural tube

dorsal gray horn

8 week embryo

Figure 1.5   Development of the spinal cord

2. Brainstem: includes the medulla oblongata, pons and midbrain

- is connected to the cerebellum conveying sensory information for control and coordination of movement
- contains sensory and motor tracts including nuclei of cranial nerves

3. Cerebellum:

- is connected to the medulla oblongata, pons and midbrain
- consists of many tracts and nuclei that influence coordination of movement, balance and posture

4. Diencephalon:

- forms the central region of the brain
- consists of the *thalamus, hypothalamus, subthalamus* and *epithalamus*
- consists of many nuclei, motor and sensory tracts.
- all sensory information, except smell, conveyed to the cerebral cortex passes through the thalamus
- the hypothalamus is important for various visceromotor functions that help maintain homeostasis

5. Cerebrum:

- consists of two cerebral hemispheres that are connected by the *corpus callosum*
- each cerebral hemisphere has many *sulci* and *gyri*
- major sulci divide each hemisphere into the frontal, parietal, temporal and occipital lobes
- each hemisphere contains many neurons and tracts. Tracts connect all cortical areas of the hemispheres as well as each hemisphere to various areas of the brain
- a large mass of gray matter, the *corpus striatum,* located at the base of each hemisphere is important in motor coordination

B. Peripheral Nervous System:

- includes 31 pairs of ***spinal nerves;*** 12 pairs of ***cranial nerves*** and the ***autonomic nervous system***
- the *autonomic nervous system* consists of two types of neurons. These are the *autonomic (visceral) sensory neurons,* that transmit information from visceral receptors to the brain and spinal cord, and the *autonomic motor neurons* that transmit information from the brain and spinal cord to smooth muscle, cardiac muscle and glands. The motor portion of the autonomic nervous system consists of two components. These are the **sympathetic** division that functions in emergency situations eg. "fight-or-flight" responses and the **parasympathetic** division that promotes less stressful activities

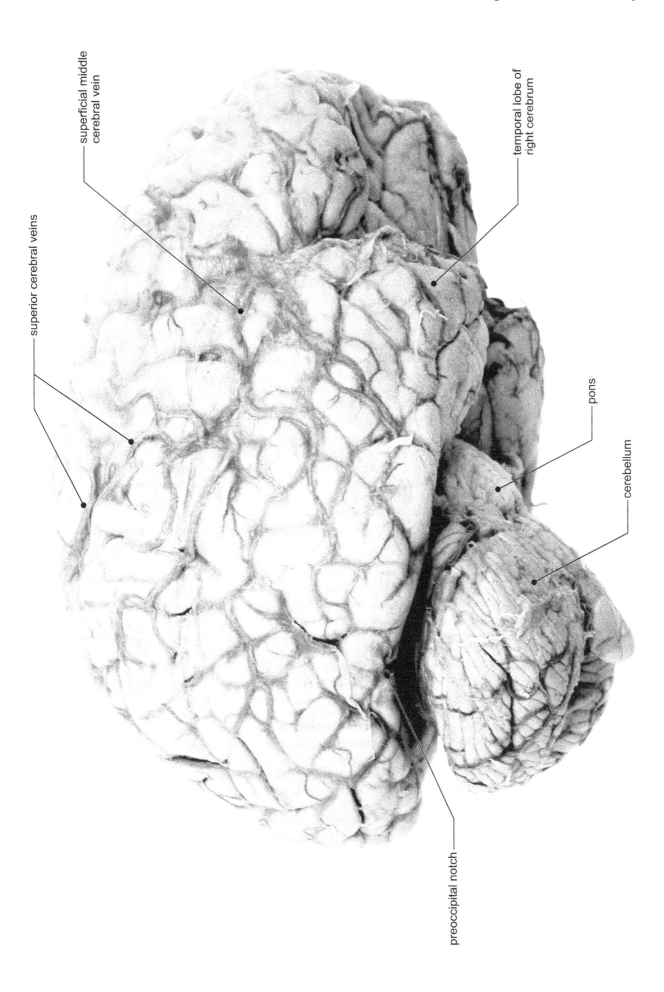

superficial middle cerebral vein

temporal lobe of right cerebrum

superior cerebral veins

pons

cerebellum

preoccipital notch

Figure 1.6   Lateral surface of the brain

CHAPTER
2

NEUROHISTOLOGY

Overview

The central nervous system consists of two major cell types, **neurons** and **neuroglial cells** or **glia.** Neurons are specialized cells that respond to stimuli from internal and external environments; process incoming information; generate new signals and conduct impulses to effectors. Neuroglial cells are supporting cells of the brain and spinal cord. The central nervous system (CNS) consists of gray matter and white matter. **Gray matter** contains cell bodies of neurons; predominantly unmyelinated axons; protoplasmic astrocytes; oligodendrocytes and microglia. In the CNS, collection of cell bodies of neurons are referred to as **nuclei** whereas those located outside the CNS are referred to as **ganglia.** The **white matter** contains predominantly myelinated axons; fibrous astrocytes; oligodendrocytes and microglia (Figure 2.1). Bundles of myelinated axons form ascending and descending **tracts**.

I. Neurons

A. Structure of Neurons:

- ranges from 5 μm to 135 μm in diameter
- most neurons have a cell body, many dendrites and one axon

1. Cell body contains:

   i. **nucleus**, with a prominent nucleolus, is located centrally and surrounded by the **cytoplasm** or **perikaryon** (Figure 2.2).

   ii. The **cytoplasm** contains:
   - **rough endoplasmic reticulum**, visualized in the light microscope as **Nissl bodies**, is involved in protein synthesis
   - **mitochondria**, involved in cellular respiration
   - **golgi apparatus,** involved in packaging and transport of protein molecules intracellularly
   - **microtubules** and **neurofilaments** are involved in cell transport
   - **lysosomes** contain enzymes that breakdown unwanted molecules
   - **lipofuscin**, a product of lysosomes, is an yellowish brown pigment that accumulates with aging. **Neuromelanin**, a black pigment present in neurons utilize catecholamines as neurotransmitters

2. Dendrites:

- are many, short, unmyelinated, branched processes that emerge from the cell body (Figure 2.2)
- dendritic branches bear small projections referred to as **dendritic spines**, which serve to increase synaptic contact
- are specialized for receiving input from the axon or cell body of the neuron

3. Axon:

- is a single process, slender, myelinated (for faster conduction of action potentials) or may be unmyelinated
- contain neurofilaments and microtubules, which are involved in transporting material to and from the cell
- cytoplasm of an axon, the **axoplasm,** is surrounded by a membrane, the **axolemma**
- is continuous with the cell body by a cone-shaped elevation, the **axon hillock** (Figure 2.2)
- the junction of the axon hillock and the point at which the axon becomes myelinated is the **initial segment**, site where several ion channels are localized and important in generating action potentials
- collateral branches may be given off from the axon
- the axon terminates by dividing into branches called **telodendria**, ending as **synaptic terminals** that contact other neurons

B. Synapses:

- are specialized regions of contact between neurons or between neurons and target cells.
- most common type of synapses are **axodendritic** and **axosomatic** (Figure 2.2); two additional types are **axoaxonal** and **dendrodendritic**.
- synapse between a motor neuron and a muscle fiber is called a **neuromuscular junction.**

1. Types of synapses:

a. **Chemical Synapses**: are polarized to conduct in one direction

   i. **Structure of a chemical synapse**:
   - **synaptic terminals** or **bouton terminal** terminate in bulb-like expansions. The plasma membrane of the synaptic terminal is thickened to form the **presynaptic membrane**
   - the cytoplasm of synaptic terminals contain numerous mitochondria and **synaptic vesicles**, which contain an inhibitory (GABA) or excitatory (glutamate) neurotransmitter. Acetylcholine is the main neurotransmitter at the neuromuscular junction, while acetylcholine and norepinephrine are important in the autonomic nervous system.

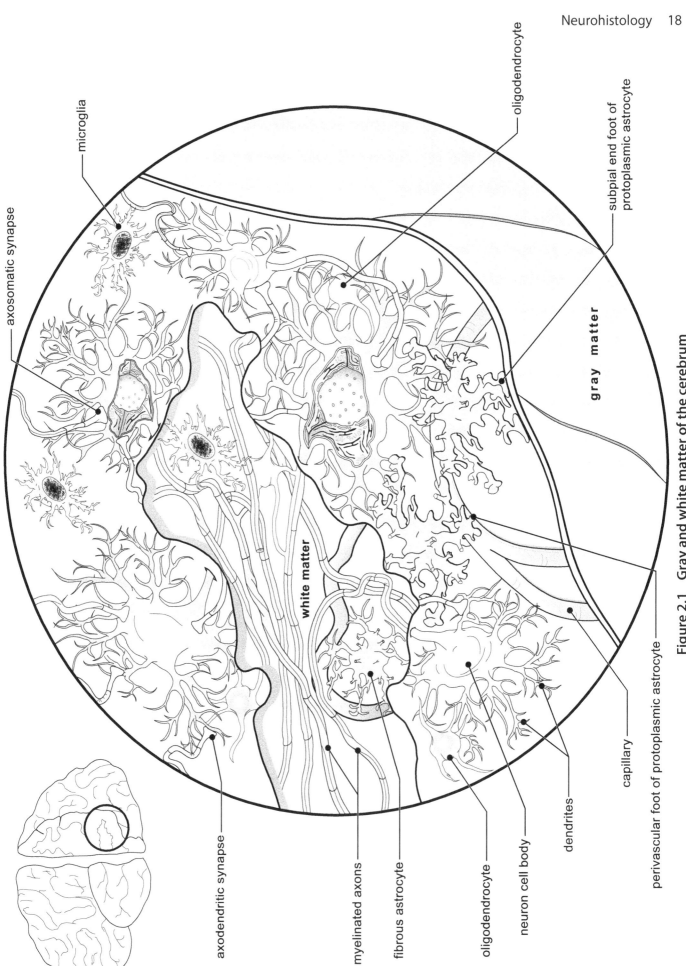

microglia

axosomatic synapse

oligodendrocyte

subpial end foot of
protoplasmic astrocyte

gray matter

white matter

axodendritic synapse

myelinated axons

fibrous astrocyte

oligodendrocyte

neuron cell body

dendrites

capillary

perivascular foot of protoplasmic astrocyte

Figure 2.1   Gray and white matter of the cerebrum

- the *postsynaptic membrane* is usually the region of the target cell membrane that receives the signal
- the extracellular space between the presynaptic membrane and postsynaptic membrane is the **synaptic cleft**

ii. *Impulse conduction across a synapse*:

action potentials arriving at a synaptic terminal $\Rightarrow$ Ca^{2+} channels open $\Rightarrow$ influx of Ca^{2+} ions $\Rightarrow$ fusion of synaptic vesicles with surface membrane of a synaptic terminal $\Rightarrow$ neurotransmitter is released via exocytosis $\Rightarrow$ binds with specific receptors on the postsynaptic membrane to initiate an excitatory or inhibitory response

b. *Electrical Synapses*: provides a low-resistance pathway and are not polarized since direction of transmission is dependent on membrane potential of cells

i. *Structure of an electrical synapse*: eg. gap junctions
- the presynaptic and postsynaptic cell membranes are closely apposed
- transmembrane proteins or *connexons* form channels that extend across and connect the cytoplasm of both cells
- electrical synapses allow passage of small ions through connexons

C. Axonal Transport:

i. *anterograde transport* – material is transported from cell body of neuron to axon terminal
- *slow anterograde* (1-5 mm/day): cytosolic proteins and components of microtubules and neurofilaments are transported along the axon for maintaining axon terminals
- *fast anterograde* (200-400 mm/day): enzymes for neurotransmitters; vesicles and mitochondria are transported at a faster rate along the axon

ii. *retrograde transport* (100 mm/day): proteins and surface molecules are transported towards the cell body of the neuron for degradation and reuse

D. Classification of Neurons:

Neurons are classified according to both structural and functional features:

1. Structural classification: based on the number of processes

a. **unipolar neurons** are sensory neurons that have a single process, which divides into a central and a peripheral branch eg. dorsal root ganglia
b. **bipolar neurons** have a single axon and a single dendrite eg. olfactory neurosensory cells
c. **multipolar neurons** have several dendrites and one axon eg. motor neurons in the brain and spinal cord (Figure 2.2)

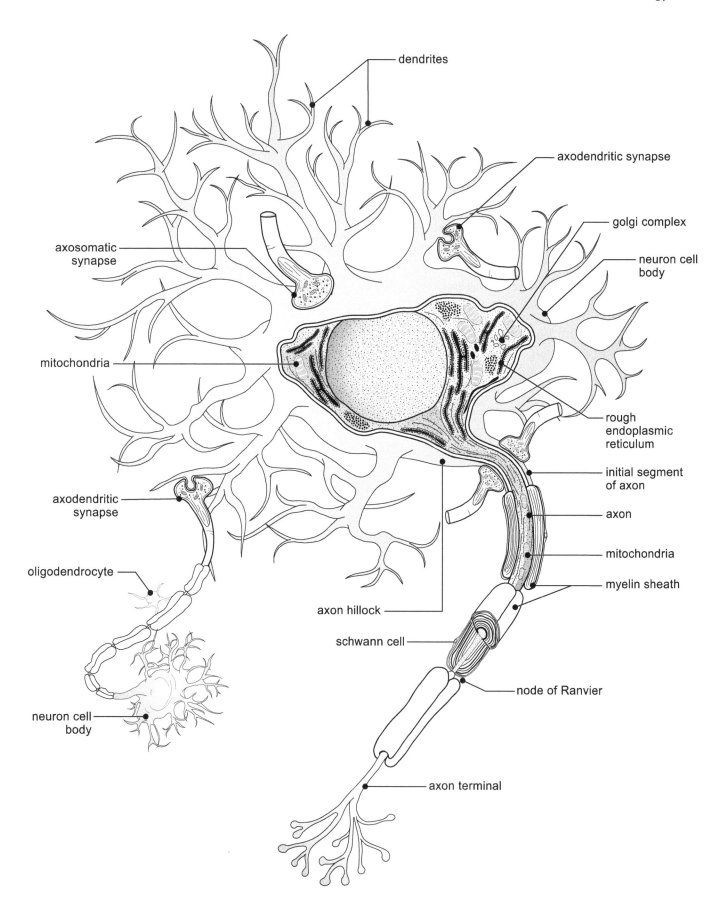

Figure 2.2 Structure of a motor neuron

2. Functional Classification:

    a. ***sensory (afferent) neurons***: transmit impulses from sensory receptors to the central nervous system. Activated sensory neurons send collaterals that excite inhibitory interneurons in the CNS, which in turn inhibit nearby sensory neurons. This is referred to as ***lateral inhibition***, that enhances central transmission while restricting transmission from peripheral areas of the receptive field

    b. ***motor (efferent) neurons***: transmit impulses from central nervous system to effectors eg. muscle; glands

    c. ***interneurons (association neurons)***: connect motor and sensory neurons and play a role in analyzing sensory information that is transmitted

II. Neuroglial Cells:

- outnumber the neurons 10:1
- do not form synapses
- have the capacity to divide
- neuroglial cells are ***astrocytes***; ***oligodendrocytes***; ***ependyma*** and ***microglia***

    a. *Astrocytes*:
- are of two types, ***fibrous*** and ***protoplasmic astrocytes***. Fibrous astrocytes occur in white matter and protoplasmic astrocytes occur in gray matter (Figure 2.1)
- are star-shaped cells with processes. Processes closely applied to capillaries form "end feet"

    functions: astrocytes function in support; in exchange of metabolites between neurons and blood (blood-brain barrier); absorption of some neurotransmitters (glutamate ions) and K^+ ions; provides insulation between synapses.

    b. *Oligodendrocytes*:
- are small cells with fewer processes
- processes of oligodendrocytes form ***myelin sheaths*** around several different axons (Figure 2.1).

    c. *Ependyma*:
- consists of ***ependymocytes*** that line the ventricular system of the brain and spinal cord, and are in contact with cerebrospinal fluid (CSF)

    d. *Microglia:*
- are elongated cells with short branched processes (Figure 2.1)
- in injury or disease, microglia are involved in phagocytosis; protection (secrete cytokines) and repair

Clinical Notes:

Degeneration and Regeneration in the Central Nervous System

A. Neuronal Reactions to Injury

- there is complete degeneration of small interneurons with injury
- injury to large neurons may affect the cell body or the axon

1. Reactions in the Cell body:

- injured neurons degenerate and reorganizational changes occur in neurons if the axon is injured
- axon injury results in changes in the cell body of the neuron, referred to as *chromatolysis*. The cell body of the neuron swells, the nucleus is displaced to an eccentric position and the Nissl bodies become granular
- degeneration of one neuron may result in *transneuronal degeneration* of the postsynaptic neuron, having been deprived of most of its afferents.

2. Reactions in the Axon:

- proximal stumps of the axon regenerate and send sprouts to the injured area of the brain or spinal cord, but growth may cease if *growth factors* that promote axonal growth are not readily available

B. Regeneration:

- mature neurons do not multiply, but functional recovery can occur after injury
- functional recovery occurs as a result of *axonal sprouting* and synapses are formed as a result of reorganization of connections by intact neurons. This is referred to as *plasticity*.

CHAPTER
3

PERIPHERAL NERVOUS SYSTEM

Overview

The Peripheral Nervous System consists of cranial and spinal nerves and the autonomic nervous system. Peripheral nerves terminate into efferent (motor) and afferent (sensory) nerve endings that link the brain and spinal cord with peripheral areas of the body. Associated with nerves are ganglia, which contain cell bodies of sensory neurons. Somatosensory information is conveyed through receptors in skin, muscles and joints

I. Spinal nerves

    a. **Roots and Rami**:

- *ventral* and *dorsal nerve roots* join to form a spinal nerve (Figure 4.2)
- there are 31 pairs of spinal nerves. These are: 8 *cervical* nerves; 12 *thoracic* nerves; 5 *lumbar* nerves; 5 *sacral* nerves and 1 *coccygeal* nerve
- spinal nerves exit at the intervertebral foramen and immediately divide into *dorsal rami* and *ventral rami*.
- *dorsal rami* supply muscles and skin of posterior neck and trunk.
- *ventral rami*, except T1 - T12, form plexuses that supply muscles and skin of the anterolateral trunk, and the upper and lower extremities.

    The major plexuses are *cervical plexus* (C1 - C4), *brachial plexus* (C4 - C8, T1) *lumbar plexus* (L1 - L4) and *sacral plexus* (S1 - S4). T1 - T12 nerves, referred to as *intercostal nerves,* supply intercostal muscles.

    b. *Functional components of spinal nerves*:

- *general somatic efferents*: supply skeletal muscles
- *general somatic afferents*: convey various sensations of touch, temperature, proprioception and pain from skin and muscles
- *general visceral afferents*: convey sensations from visceral organs
- *general visceral efferents*: supply viscera (smooth muscle, glands etc.) via the autonomic nervous system

II. Types of Receptors:

i. sensory nerve endings in skin that respond to touch, pressure, vibration are ***exteroceptors***; those that respond to pain are ***nociceptors*** and those that respond to temperature are ***thermoreceptors***

ii. sensory nerve endings in muscles, tendons and joints that respond to joint position and movement are ***proprioceptors***

iii. sensory nerve endings in viscera and blood vessels are ***interoceptors***

III. Distribution:

A. Sensory Innervation:

- parallel segments of the skin are innervated by a single spinal nerve. Each segment of skin is a **dermatome**. Each nerve supplies its own segment and half of each adjacent segment. Knowledge of the segmental innervation of the skin is important for detecting the level of lesion of the spinal cord or nerve roots.

i. Cutaneous Receptors:

Receptors occur as free nerve endings or are encapsulated. Distribution of various receptors present in the epidermis and dermis of the skin are indicated in Figure 3.1. These are:
- ***meissner's corpuscle***: responds to light touch and pressure
- ***merkel endings***: detects discriminative touch
- ***ruffini ending***: detects pressure
- ***pacinian corpuscle***: responds to vibration
- ***free nerve endings:*** detects pain and temperature

ii. Receptors in joints and muscles (proprioceptors):

Refer to Figure 3.2. These are:

a. **muscle spindle**: monitor changes in length of muscle and have both a motor and a sensory innervation

- consists of a capsule enclosing 6 to 10 **intrafusal fibers** that are surrounded by **extrafusal fibers**
- there are two types of intrafusal fibers. The nuclear bag fiber has all the nuclei arranged in the middle part of the fiber. In the nuclear chain fiber, nuclei are evenly distributed along the muscle fiber
- intrafusal fibers are contractile only at their ends and are supplied by **gamma motor neurons**
- the noncontractile central part of intrafusal fibers are innervated by afferent type la and type ll nerve fibers. Thus, when the muscle lengthens, the muscle spindle is stretched resulting in depolarization of the afferent fibers

b. *golgi tendon organ*: detects tension and force of muscle contraction applied to a tendon

- is located at the junction of a tendon and muscle
- consists of a thin capsule enclosing few collagen fibers
- is innervated by afferent type lb fibers

B. Motor innervation of skeletal muscle:

i. motor fibers enter a muscle as a unit, referred to as the ***neuromuscular junction***.

The structure of the neuromuscular junction is as follows:

- the axon loses the myelin sheath as it reaches the muscle fiber and ends by forming ***terminals*** or ***boutons*** that are located in a depression on the surface of the muscle fiber and separated by the ***synaptic cleft***
- nerve terminals contain mitochondria and ***synaptic vesicles*** that contain acetylcholine
- the underlying sarcolemma is arranged into junctional folds containing ***acetylcholine receptors***
- action potentials propagated along the axon triggers release of acetylcholine by exocytosis
- acetylcholine binds with acetylcholine receptors in the postsynaptic membrane resulting in initiation of muscle contraction

ii. Skeletal muscles are innervated by ***alpha*** and ***gamma motor neurons***. Alpha motor neurons innervate extrafusal muscle fibers and gamma motor neurons innervate intrafusal muscle fibers of neuromuscular spindles. Skeletal muscles are innervated by more than one spinal nerve. Muscles innervated by a spinal cord segment constitutes a ***myotome***. Innervation of muscles can be tested by muscle reflexes eg. biceps tendon reflex (C5, C6); patellar tendon reflex (L3, L4); calcaneal tendon reflex (S1, S2).

A motor neuron, its axon and all the muscle fibers it innervates is a ***motor unit***. Muscles of the eye have fewer number of muscle fibers to a motor unit and are capable of more precise control. In contrast, muscles of the back have about 1000 muscle fibers to a motor unit. All muscle fibers in a motor unit are of the same type and contract simultaneously when stimulated. Larger diameter, faster-conducting alpha motor neurons innervate fast twitch muscle fibers while smaller diameter, slower-conducting alpha motor neurons innervate slow twitch muscle fibers. Thus, there are fast-twitch motor units and slow twitch motor units. At the initiation of muscle contraction small motor units are recruited first, and with increasing force larger ones are recruited. Even at rest, some motor units are active, this resting tension in a muscle is referred to as ***muscle tone***. Muscle tone is controlled by afferent nerve endings in a muscle and is dependent on the integrity of the monosynaptic stretch reflex.

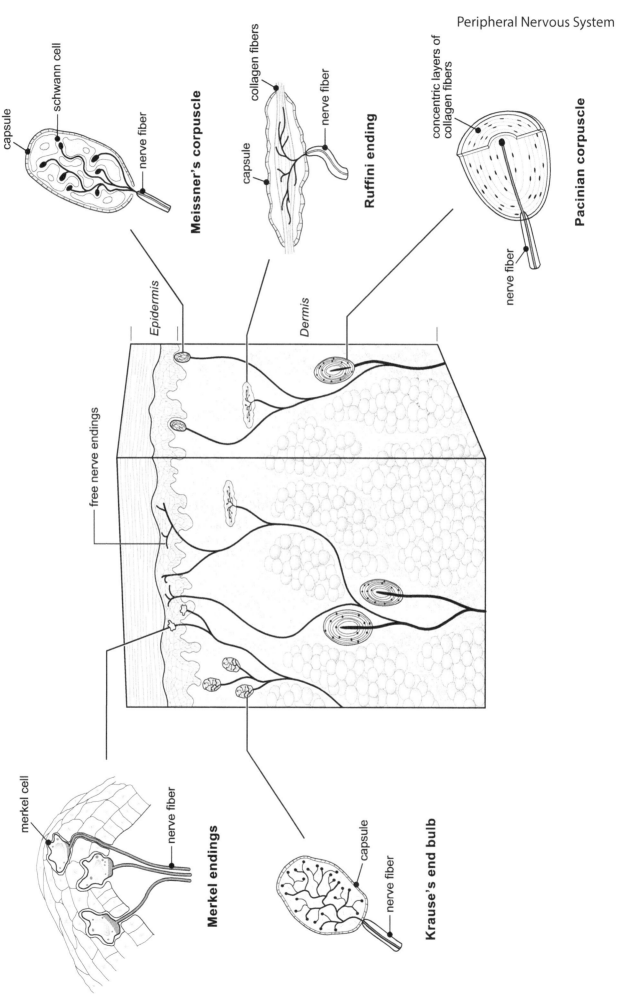

Figure 3.1   Sensory receptors in skin

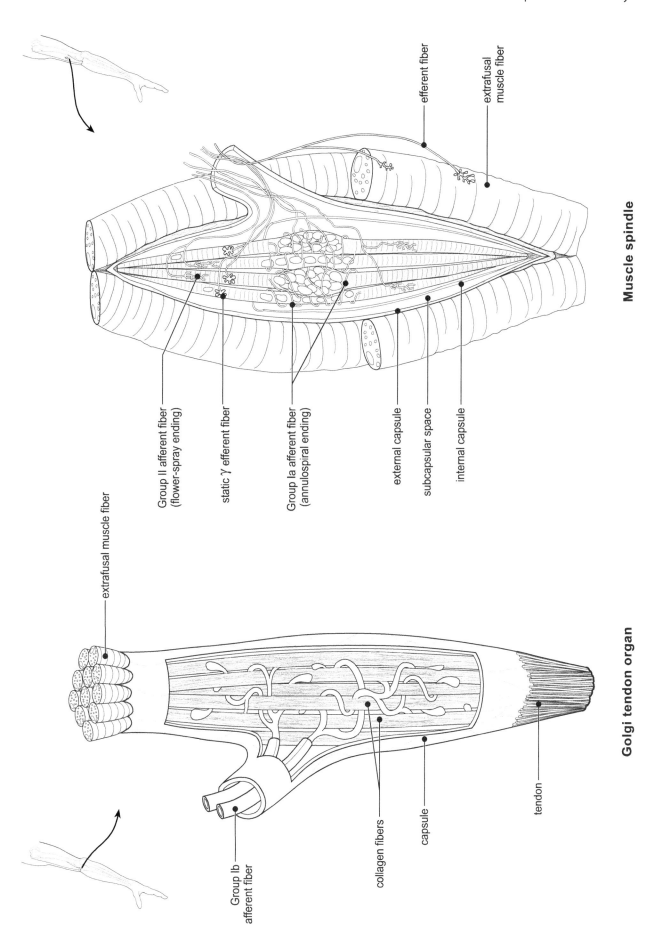

Muscle spindle

efferent fiber

extrafusal
muscle fiber

Group II afferent fiber
(flower-spray ending)

static γ efferent fiber

Group Ia afferent fiber
(annulospiral ending)

external capsule

subcapsular space

internal capsule

extrafusal muscle fiber

Golgi tendon organ

Group Ib
afferent fiber

collagen fibers

capsule

tendon

Figure 3.2   Muscle proprioceptors

Clinical Notes:

a. **Myasthenia gravis**: is an autoimmune disease that affects synaptic transmission at the neuromuscular junction. In this disease, antibodies to acetylcholine receptors are produced. Antibodies bind to acetylcholine receptors, blocking the normal action of acetylcholine at the neuromuscular junction.

b. Pathological changes in muscle tone result in diseases of the nervous system. **Hypotonia** (or **flaccidity**) involves decreased or loss of muscle tone. Muscles appear loose and flattened. Hypotonia occurs in cerebellar disorders and lower motor neuron lesions. **Hypertonia** or increased muscle tone, can be either **spastic** or **rigid**. **Spasticity** is a condition in which there is increased resistance to rapid stretching of muscles due to abnormal activity of the stretch reflexes, which is normally suppressed by the descending motor tracts. Hyperactive stretch reflexes can also show **clonus**, which consists of rhythmic contractions and relaxations that are elicited when a tendon is stretched. **Rigidity** is increased muscle tone that occurs with very slow, passive movements, as in Parkinson's disease or upper motor neuron lesions . In" **clasp-knife rigidity**" there is sudden decrease in resistance when a flexed joint is rapidly extended. This effect is to due an inhibitory reflex initiated by the golgi tendon organs, resulting in a sudden relaxation of the muscles.

IV. Peripheral Nerves:

Peripheral nerves are bundles of nerve fibers surrounded by several connective tissue sheaths. Refer to Table 3.1 for classification and types of nerve fibers

a. *Connective tissue sheaths* (Figure 4.2)

- *epineurium*: outermost connective tissue sheath that cover nerves
- *perineurium*: collagen fibers and flattened cells that cover bundles of nerve fibers provide a barrier to macromolecules and protects nerve fibers
- *endoneurium*: loose connective tissue covering a nerve fiber (axon)

b. **Nerve Fiber:**

- consists of an axon with or without a ***myelin sheath*** and the ensheathing glial cell. Axons with a myelin sheath are **myelinated.** Axons without such a covering are **unmyelinated**.
- two types of cells, the ***schwann cell*** and the ***oligodendrocyte***, produce myelin sheaths. The ***schwann cells*** of the peripheral nervous system, myelinates only one axon. Each process of an **oligodendrocyte,** in the central nervous system, myelinates different axons.

- the myelin sheath , a multilayered covering, begins just distal to the origin of the axon and ends before the axon terminates into *axon terminals* or *telodendria* (Figure 2.2).
- the schwann cell (or oligodendrocyte) wraps around the axon. The inner layers of the schwann cell fuses and wraps around the nerve fiber to form the myelin sheath, a lipoprotein complex. The myelin sheath protect axons and maintain a constant ionic microenvironment for conduction of action potentials.
- junctions along the myelin sheath are referred to as *nodes of Ranvier* (Figure 2.2). Action potentials jump from node to node, referred to as **saltatory conduction**.
- the largest axons have thicker myelin sheaths and greater external diameters. The greater the diameter of a nerve fiber, the faster the conduction velocity of an impulse.
- *unmyelinated fibers* are slow, small diameter fibers that are surrounded by glial cell membranes but lack myelin sheaths. Many unmyelinated axons are ensheathed by a single schwann cell.

b. **Peripheral Nerve Injuries and Disorders:**

Pathological processes in nerves involve motor and sensory deficits. Contributing factors to nerve lesions are:
- *degenerative disc disease* may lead to impingement on a spinal nerve roots, usually at C6 - C7 or L5 - S1 levels.
- *tumors* involving nerve roots or meninges can cause compression and pain
- *spinal canal stenosis* or narrowing of the spinal canal can cause nerve compression
- *facet syndrome:* bony spurs that form around the facet joints of the vertebrae cause narrowing of the spinal canal with inflammation and compression of nerve roots

Table 3.1 Classification of Receptors and Types of Nerve Fibers

TYPE OF NERVE FIBER	TYPE OF RECEPTOR	FUNCTION
SOMATIC EFFERENTS		
Aα (alpha motor neurons)		motor to skeletal muscle (extrafusal fibers)
Aγ (gamma motor neurons)		motor to muscle spindle (intrafusal muscle fibers)
MUSCLE & CUTANEOUS AFFERENTS *Myelinated fibers*		
1a	Muscle spindles (annulospiral endings)	muscle stretch
1b	Golgi tendon organs	tendon tension
II **Aβ**	Muscle spindles (flower-spray endings) Meissner's corpuscle Pacinian corpuscle	muscle stretch, touch, vibration proprioception
Aδ or III	Free nerve endings	pain, temperature
Unmyelinated fibers		
C or IV	Free nerve endings	pain, temperature

A few examples of peripheral nerve lesions are:

i. ***Radiculopathy*** or compression syndromes:

Compression of a spinal nerve root results in ***radicular*** or ***'girdle' pain*** in the distribution of a dermatome. The most common cause is ***spondylosis*** or disease of the intervertebral disc, which is common for C6, C7, L5 and S1 nerve roots.

a. *Sciatica*: compression of S1 nerve root by a herniated intervertebral disc

> Symptoms: are numbness in the posterior thigh and leg, lateral border of the foot and 4-5 toes with weakness of plantar flexion and eversion of the foot

b. *Radial nerve palsy*: compression of the radial nerve as a result of prolonged pressure of the shaft of the humerus.

> Symptoms: are sensory loss over posterior forearm and dorsum of the hand; loss of extension of forearm, wrist and hand; loss of supination of forearm resulting in "**wrist drop**"

ii. *Entrapment syndromes*: occurs when a nerve is compressed as it runs through a narrow space.

a. *carpal tunnel syndrome*: the median nerve can be compressed as it runs below the flexor retinaculum through the carpal tunnel at the wrist.

> Symptoms: are pain, numbness in 1-3 fingers, weakness of abduction, flexion and opposition of the thumb.

b. *thoracic outlet syndrome:* compression of the upper trunk of the brachial plexus by a cervical rib or by the scalenus anterior muscle. The upper trunk of the brachial plexus, the *Erb's* type of paralysis, involves C5, C6 roots.

> Symptoms: are weakness of shoulder abduction, forearm flexion, and wrist extension. As a result, the upper limb is extended, adducted and medially rotated with the forearm pronated and fingers flexed. The upper limb assumes the "waiter's tip" position.

c. *Ulnar nerve palsy*: entrapment of the ulnar nerve at the elbow or compression of the nerve in the palm at the narrow ulnar carpal canal (canal of *Guyon*), located between the pisiform bone proximally and the hook of the hamate medially.

> Symptoms: are pain; numbness of medial side of palm and 4-5 fingers; weak wrist adduction; loss of adduction and abduction of fingers; loss of flexion at metacarpophalangeal joints and extension at interphalangeal joints, referred to as *claw hand*.

d. *Meralgia paraesthetica:* entrapment of the lateral femoral cutaneous nerve (originating from L2 and L3) near the anterior superior iliac spine as it passes below the inguinal ligament.

Symptoms: are burning or tingling sensation over the anterolateral thigh. There is no motor involvement.

e. *Peroneal nerve palsy:* entrapment of the common peroneal nerve at the neck of fibula.

Symptoms: are numbness of the lateral aspect of the leg and dorsum of foot; weak dorsiflexion and eversion of foot resulting in "foot drop" and high steppage gait (knee raised high at each step)

iii. *Denervation*:

a. Axons and dendrites may be repaired if the neuron cell body remains intact. Degeneration of the distal segment of an axon is referred to as *Wallerian degeneration*. Changes that occur distal to the site of injury are as follows:

- axon and myelin sheath break down
- phagocytic cells invade the area and remove cellular debris
- distal stump of the nerve is filled with tubular structures and schwann cells, referred to as **bands of von Bungner**

b. Axonal regeneration in severed nerves:

- macrophages and fibroblasts fill the interval between cut ends of the nerve
- schwann cells and regenerating axons invade the area
- the proximal segment of each axon divides into many branches and the enlarged tip of each branch form *growth cones*
- each branch invades a single *bands of von Bungner* of the distal segment of the axon
- axonal branches grow along the interval between schwann cells and the basal lamina, resulting in regeneration of the injured nerve.
- axonal branches that grow in random directions and fail to connect with the distal segment form a painful disorganized swelling or *neuroma.* Neuromas formed at the stump of an amputed limb are thought to be the main cause of **phantom limb pain**.

CHAPTER
4

SPINAL CORD

Overview

The spinal cord is a continuation of the brainstem. In the spinal cord the gray matter is centrally located and is surrounded by the white matter. The gray matter consists of cell bodies of neurons and dendrites. The white matter is organized into bundles of nerve fibers or ascending and descending tracts that have a similar function. Tracts are grouped into columns that extend the whole length of the cord. Thirty-one spinal nerves connect on each side of the cord, serving as a link for transmission of impulses between the brain and various areas of the body. The spinal cord is also important for integration of reflex activity.

I. Gross Anatomy:

A. Location:

- located in the vertebral canal
- extends from foramen magnum to junction of L1 and L2

B. Coverings:

1. **pia mater**: innermost, thin fibrous layer that adheres to the surface of the spinal cord (Figure 4.1).

2. **arachnoid mater**: middle, thin layer of connective tissue. Between the arachnoid mater and the pia mater is the **subarachnoid space** that contains cerebrospinal fluid. The subarachnoid space caudal to the termination of the cord, referred to as the *lumbar cistern*, contains the lumbosacral nerve roots

3. **dura mater**: is the thick superficial fibrous layer, continuous with the dura mater of the brain. Between the dura mater and the arachnoid mater is the **subdural space.** Between the dura mater and the vertebral canal is the **epidural space,** which contains fat and plexus of veins. Projections of the arachnoid mater and pia mater form the **denticulate ligaments** that suspend the cord in the dural sheath (Figure 4.1)

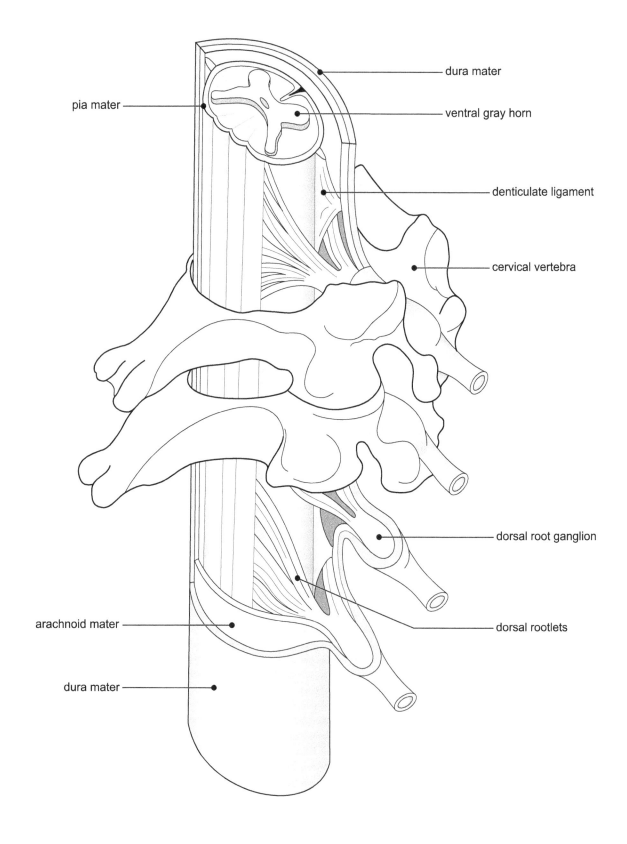

pia mater

dura mater

ventral gray horn

denticulate ligament

cervical vertebra

dorsal root ganglion

arachnoid mater

dorsal rootlets

dura mater

Figure 4.1   Meninges of the spinal cord

C. Features

1. **External Features:**

   - long, cylindrical structure
   - the cord ends as a cone-like structure, the **conus medullaris** (Figure 4.2)
   - the conus medullaris tapers into a thin filament, the *filum terminale* (Figure 4.2) The filum terminale is comprised of pia mater and dura mater and attaches the cord to the coccyx
   - lumbosacral nerve roots (L3 - Co1) surround the filum terminale and constitute the **cauda equina**
   - the external surface of the cord is divided into ventral, lateral and dorsal areas by longitudinal grooves. The **ventral** (**anterior**) **median fissure** is a deep groove on the ventral surface and contains the anterior spinal artery. The **dorsal median sulcus** is a shallow groove on the dorsal surface of the cord

2. *Limb Enlargements*:

   i.   **cervical enlargement** includes C4 - T1 segments of cord. Spinal nerves from these segments form the brachial plexus for innervation of the upper limbs
   ii. **lumbosacral enlargement** is located distally and includes L2 - S3 segments of cord. Spinal nerves from these segments form the lumbosacral plexus for innervation of the lower limbs.

3. *Spinal segments*:

   - there are 31 pairs of spinal nerves
   - each pair of spinal nerve arises from a segment of the spinal cord (Figure 4.2).
   - there are *31 segments* of the spinal cord

4. *Roots:*

   a. *dorsal root:* composed of rootlets along each segment of the cord (Figure 4.2) and is segregated into *lateral* and *medial divisions* as it enters the cord.
   b. *ventral root:* arises by rootlets along each segment of the cord
   c. *spinal nerves:* are formed by ventral and dorsal roots.

   There are: *cervical nerves (C1–C8); thoracic nerves, (T1–T12); lumbar nerves (L1–L5); sacral nerves (S1–S5) and coccygeal nerve (Co1).*

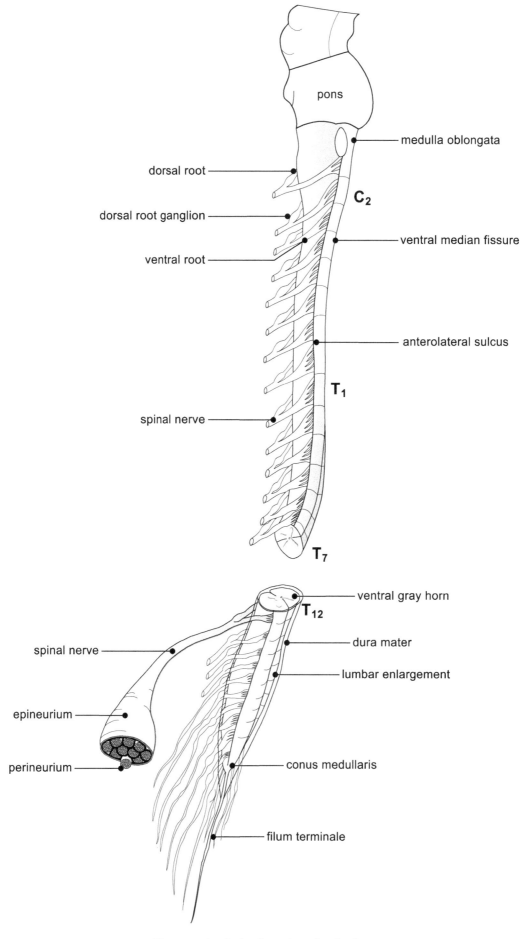

pons

medulla oblongata

dorsal root

C₂

dorsal root ganglion

ventral median fissure

ventral root

anterolateral sulcus

T₁

spinal nerve

T₇

ventral gray horn

T₁₂

spinal nerve

dura mater

lumbar enlargement

epineurium

perineurium

conus medullaris

filum terminale

Figure 4.2   Spinal cord and spinal nerves

5. *Internal Features*: consists of gray matter and white matter

    a. **Gray matter:** is centrally located, H-shaped and surrounded by the white matter (Figure 4.3). It is subdivided in each half of the cord as indicated in Figures 4.3 and 4.4. These are:

        i. *dorsal gray horn*: consisting mainly of ***tract cells*** and ***interneurons***
        ii. *intermediate zone*: consisting of ***interneurons*** and ***neurons***
        iii. *ventral gray horn*: consists of ***alpha motor neurons*** and ***gamma motor neurons***
        iv. *lateral gray horn:* present in the thoracic and upper lumbar segments of the cord. It consists of preganglionic neurons of the ***autonomic nervous system***.
        v. The ***gray commissure*** forms the crossbar of the "H". In the center is the ***central canal***. It extends the entire length of the spinal cord and contains cerebrospinal fluid.

    b. **White matter:** consists of three *funiculi* as indicated in Figures 4.5 to 4.8 These are:

        i. *dorsal funiculi*: consists of the ***fasciculus gracilis*** that extends throughout the length of the cord. Above the midthoracic level, the ***fasciculus cuneatus*** is also present, and is located lateral to the fasciculus gracilis
        ii. *lateral funiculi*: consists of ascending and descending tracts
        iii. *ventral funiculi*: consists of ascending and descending tracts

    c. *Dorsolateral tract* (***tract of Lissauer***) occupies the area between the surface of the spinal cord and apex of the dorsal gray horn. Dorsal root afferents conveying pain and temperature enter the spinal cord by way of the dorsolateral tract, where they ascend or descend for short distances, giving off branches that enter the dorsal gray horn

D. Organization of Gray matter and White matter:

1. **Gray matter:** Neurons are arranged longitudinally into columns or nuclei and can be subdivided into 10 laminae, referred to as ***laminae of Rexed***. Distribution of laminae vary at different segmental levels of the spinal cord, but typical cross sections at the cervical, thoracic, lumbar and sacral levels are shown in Figures 4.5 to 4.8.

    a. *Dorsal gray horn:* includes ***laminae 1 - V1***. Dorsal root afferents end in the dorsal gray horn (Figure 4.3).

      • *lamina 1* is a thin layer that consists mainly of interneurons and dorsal root afferents conveying pain, temperature and touch sensations
      • *lamina 11*, located below *lamina 1* is the ***substantia gelatinosa***. Neurons of the substantia gelatinosa receive thin myelinated and unmyelinated afferents that convey pain, temperature and touch information and play a role in modulation of pain

- *lamina 111* consists of interneurons and dorsal root afferents
- *lamina 1V* contains *tract cells,* whose axons cross the midline and ascend in the contralateral spinothalamic tract (Figure 4.3).
- *lamina V* and *lamina V1* are located at the base of the dorsal gray horn. This zone consists of *tract cells* and interneurons. Lamina 1V, V and V1 are collectively referred to as *nucleus proprius*.

b. **Intermediate Zone**: occupies the area between the dorsal gray horn and ventral gray horn, including the space within the ventral gray horn. It includes *lamina V11*.

- *lamina V11* consists of *interneurons* and *nuclei* (cell columns). The cell columns are:

    i. *nucleus thoracicus (nucleus dorsalis)*
        - is located in the thoracic and upper lumbar spinal segments (Figure 4.4). Axons of neurons in nucleus thoracicus (*T1–L3*) form the *dorsal spinocerebellar tract*

    ii. *intermediolateral cell column*:
        - are preganglionic sympathetic neurons in the lateral gray horn
        - is located in the thoracic and upper lumbar spinal segments (*T1–L3*)

    iii. *sacral autonomic nucleus*
        - are preganglionic parasympathetic neurons, in the lateral part of lamina V11
        - is located in the sacral spinal segments (*S2–S4*)

c. **Ventral gray horn:** includes laminae V11 - 1X (Figure 4.4)

- *lamina V111* is located on the medial side of the ventral gray horn. Many descending tracts terminate in lamina V111
- *lamina 1X* consists of large *alpha motor neurons*; groups of smaller *gamma motor neurons* and *interneurons (Renshaw cells)* interspersed between groups of alpha motor neurons. Alpha motor neurons supply skeletal muscles. In general, alpha motor neurons that supply *axial muscles* are located medially (medial cell column) in the ventral gray horn, while those that supply *limb muscles* are located laterally (lateral cell column) in the ventral gray horn of the cervical and lumbosacral enlargements of the cord. Motor neurons supplying proximal muscles (shoulder and hip) are located more ventrally than motor neurons that supply distal muscles (hand and foot). Gamma motor neurons supply intrafusal fibers of muscle spindles
- the cervical cord also contains the *phrenic nucleus* (supplies the *diaphragm*) and *spinal accessory nucleus* (supplies the trapezius and sternocleidomastoid).
- *lamina X* surrounds the central canal of the spinal cord.

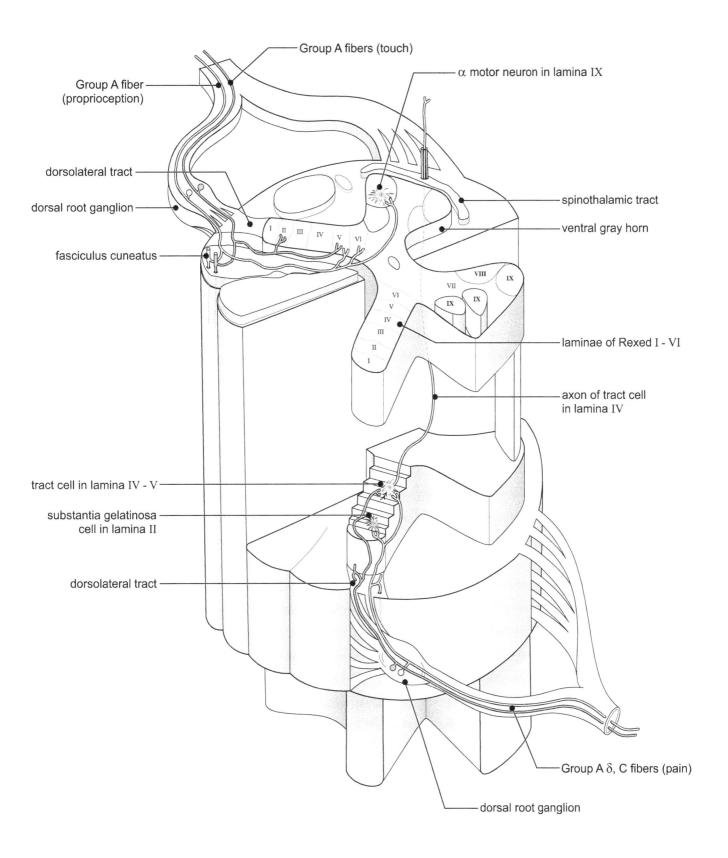

Figure 4.3   Circuitry of the dorsal gray horn of the spinal cord

d. **Neuronal circuitry**:

  i. *Dorsal gray horn*:

- information from sensory receptors enter the spinal cord by way of the dorsal roots. The cell bodies of sensory neurons are located in the dorsal root ganglion. Dorsal root afferents are divided into lateral and medial divisions as they enter the cord.
Refer to Figure 4.3 for the circuitry of the dorsal gray horn.
- the *lateral division of dorsal root*, contains thin myelinated (Group Aδ) or unmyelinated (Group C) fibers conveying pain, temperature and touch sensations. Fibers enter the *dorsolateral tract of Lissauer*, divide into ascending and descending branches and synapse with interneurons and tract cells of the dorsal gray horn
- the *medial division of dorsal root* containing large myelinated afferents (Group A) convey proprioception and vibration. Fibers enter the dorsal funiculus, divide into ascending and descending branches and terminate in the dorsal gray horn.

  ii. *Ventral gray horn:* consists of motor neurons and interneurons (Figure 4.4).

    a. Motor neurons are:

- *alpha motor neurons* supply extrafusal fibers of skeletal muscles. Output of alpha motor neurons is regulated by inhibitory interneurons, the **Renshaw cells**. Renshaw cells make inhibitory synapses on alpha motor neurons and also receives excitatory synapses from collaterals of the same alpha motor neurons. Alpha motor neurons that are excitatory activate Renshaw cells, which in turn, inhibit the activity of the same alpha motor neurons. Thus by inhibiting nearby motor neurons, activation of frequently firing motor neurons are maintained.
- *gamma motor neurons* - supply intrafusal fibers of skeletal muscles
- motor neurons of the spinal cord are collectively referred to as *lower motor neurons* compared to motor neurons of the cerebral cortex and brain stem which are *upper motor neurons.*

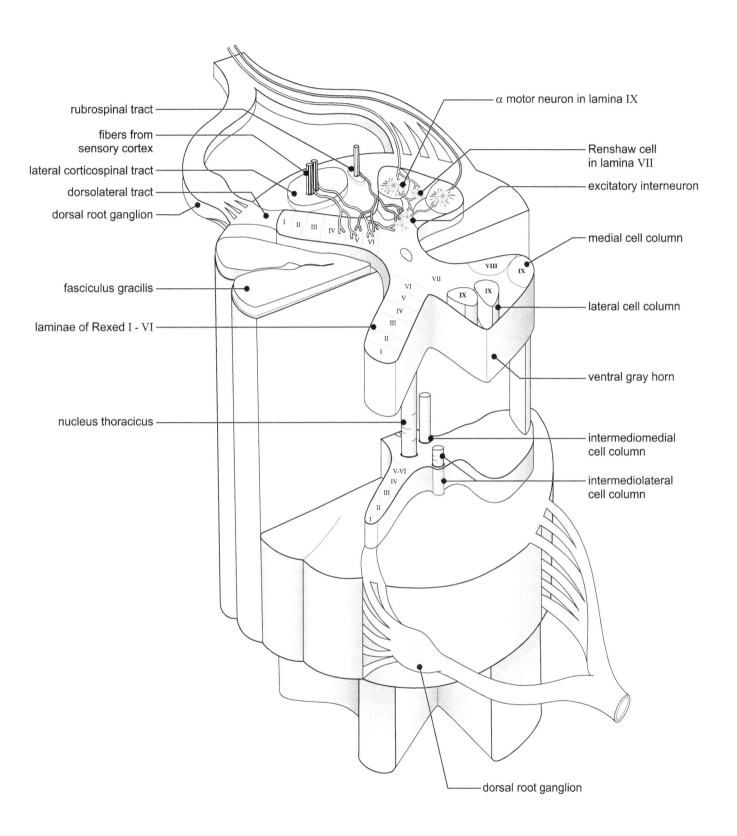

Figure 4.4 Circuitry of the ventral gray horn of the spinal cord

2. **White Matter of the Spinal cord**:

- consists of the *dorsal*, *lateral* and *ventral funiculi.*
- *dorsal funiculi* contain two ascending tracts
- the *lateral* and *ventral funiculi* contain ascending and descending tracts
- sensory fibers enter the dorsal funiculus on the lateral side of the cord. An orderly arrangement, or *somatotopic organization* results, with the sacral fibers located most medial and the cervical fibers located most lateral as they ascend the cord.

Refer to Figures 4.5 to 4.8 for the various tracts in cross sections at the cervical, thoracic, lumbar and sacral levels of the spinal cord.

a. *Dorsal funiculus* - contains the *medial lemniscus system* (**posterior** or *dorsal columns*) that convey *fine touch; proprioception* and *vibratory sense* from the upper and lower limbs.

The *Medial Lemniscus System* consists of the *fasciculus gracilis* and *fasciculus cuneatus* (Table 4.1)

Table 4.1 The Medial Lemniscus System

TRACT	ORIGIN	TERMINATION	FUNCTION
Fasciculus gracilis	dorsal root ganglion (primary neuron)	nucleus gracilis (ipsilateral)	fine touch, proprioception, vibration from contralateral lower limbs
Fasciculus cuneatus	dorsal root ganglion (primary neuron)	nucleus cuneatus (ipsilateral)	fine touch, proprioception, vibration from contralateral upper limbs

b. **Lateral funiculus**: consists of descending and ascending tracts (Tables 4.2 and 4.3)

Table 4.2 Descending tracts in the lateral funiculus of the spinal cord

TRACT	ORIGIN	TERMINATION	FUNCTION
Lateral corticospinal tract	primary motor area, premotor area and primary sensory area	lamina 1V - V11 and 1X of spinal cord (contralateral)	control of skilled movements
Rubrospinal tract	red nucleus	lamina V11; 1X of spinal cord (contralateral)	control of movement
Raphespinal tract	nucleus raphe magnus	lamina 1-111 of spinal cord (ipsilateral)	modulates pain

Table 4.3 Ascending tracts in the lateral funiculus of the spinal cord

TRACT	ORIGIN	TERMINATION	FUNCTION
Dorsal spinocerebellar tract	nucleus thoracicus	cerebellum (ipsilateral)	unconscious proprioception (lower limbs) for coordination of movement
Ventral spinocerebellar tract	dorsal gray horn of lumbosacral segments of cord (contralateral)	cerebellum	unconscious proprioception (lower limbs) for coordination of movement
Spinothalamic tract	laminae 1V, V-V1 of dorsal gray horn	primary sensory cortex (contralateral)	pain, touch and temperature
Spinoreticular tract	laminae 1V - V111 of dorsal gray horn	medullary reticular formation (ipsilateral) and pontine reticular formation (contralateral)	consciousness and alertness, pain
Spinomesencephalic (Spinotectal) tract	dorsal gray horn	superior colliculus (contralateral)	coordination of head and eye movements

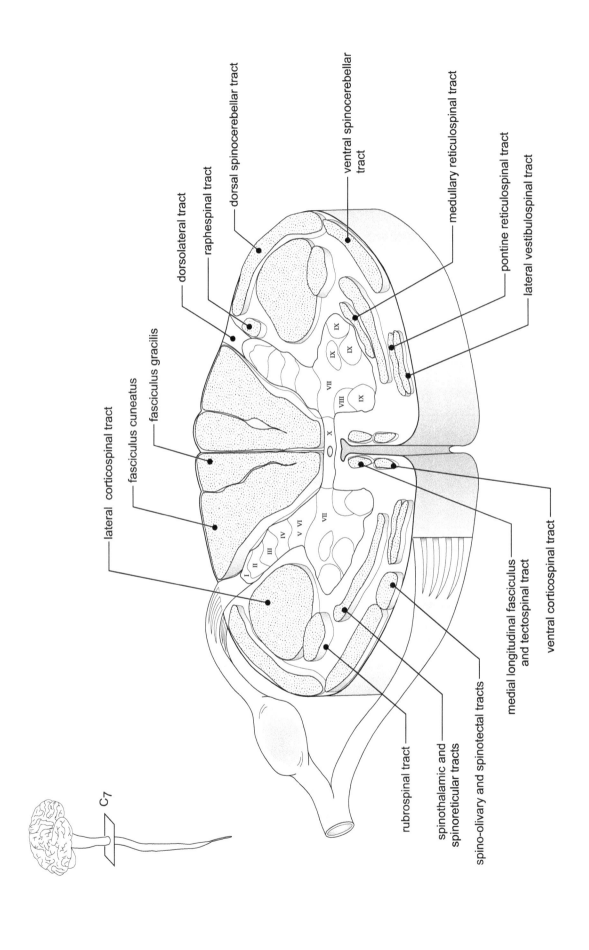

dorsal spinocerebellar tract

raphespinal tract

dorsolateral tract

fasciculus gracilis

fasciculus cuneatus

lateral corticospinal tract

ventral spinocerebellar tract

medullary reticulospinal tract

pontine reticulospinal tract

lateral vestibulospinal tract

rubrospinal tract

spinothalamic and spinoreticular tracts

spino-olivary and spinotectal tracts

medial longitudinal fasciculus and tectospinal tract

ventral corticospinal tract

C₇

Figure 4.5   Cross section of the cervical cord

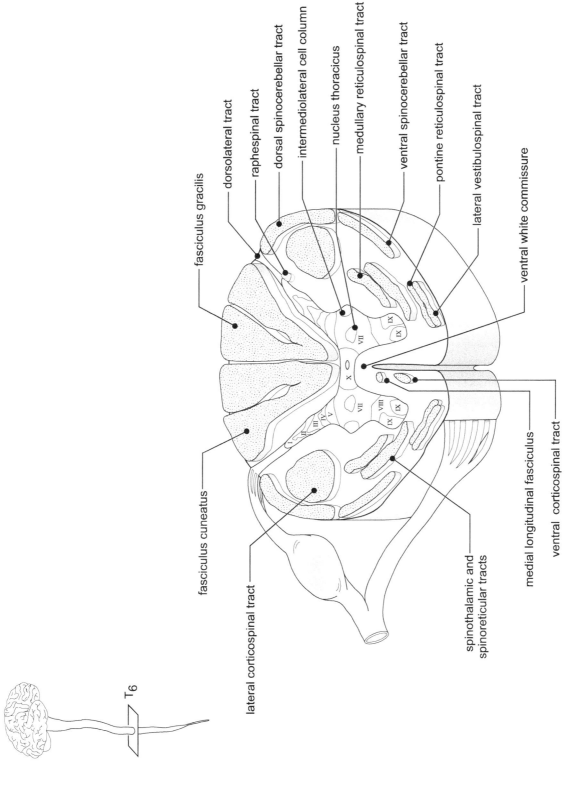

Figure 4.6   Cross section of the thoracic cord

c. **Ventral funiculus:** consists of descending tracts (Table 4.4)

Table 4.4 Tracts in the ventral funiculus of the spinal cord

TRACT	ORIGIN	TERMINATION	FUNCTION
Ventral corticospinal tract	primary motor area; premotor area and primary sensory area	uncrossed in medulla but crosses at segmental spinal levels, terminating in laminae 1V - V11; 1X	control of trunk and shoulder girdle muscles
Lateral vestibulospinal tract	lateral vestibular nucleus	laminae V11,V111 and 1X of spinal cord (ipsilateral)	control of posture
Medial longitudinal fasciculus (Medial vestibulospinal tract)	medial vestibular nucleus	upper cervical levels of the spinal cord (bilateral)	coordinates head and eye movements
Reticulospinal tract	reticular formation (central group of reticular nuclei in pons and medulla)	laminae VII - IX of spinal cord (ipsilateral/bilateral)	control of movements of limbs
Tectospinal tract	superior colliculus	upper cervical segments of cord (contralateral)	head movements in response to visual stimuli

E. Spinal Reflexes: are automatic responses to changes in the environment

1. *Stretch Reflex:* is a monosynaptic reflex. The circuitry is indicated in Figure 4.9 and summarized using the patellar reflex as an example.

    A quick tap to the patellar tendon stretches the quadriceps femoris tendon resulting in stimulation of muscle spindles → impulses conveyed via *1a* afferents → afferent neurons in dorsal root ganglion → via dorsal root → dorsal gray horn → alpha motor neurons that innervate extrafusal fibers of quadriceps femoris → contraction of quadriceps femoris muscle

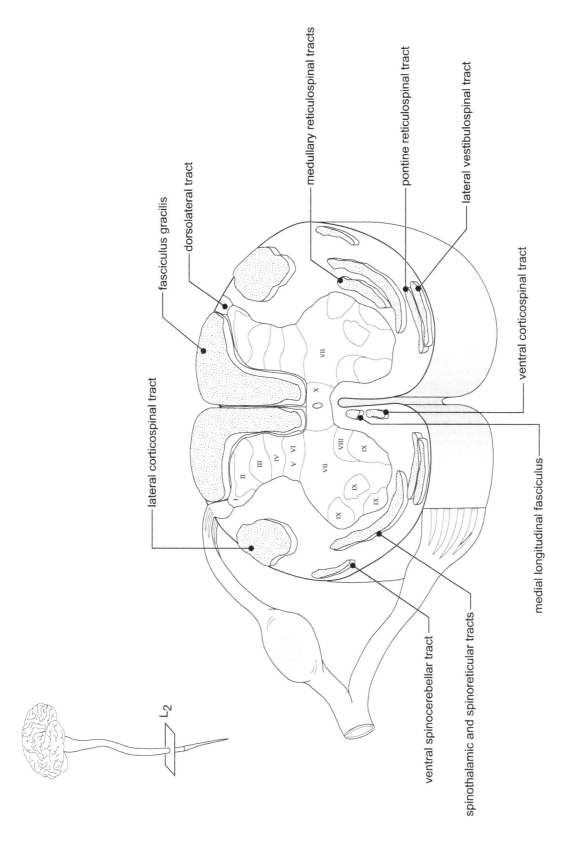

Figure 4.7   Cross section of the lumbar cord

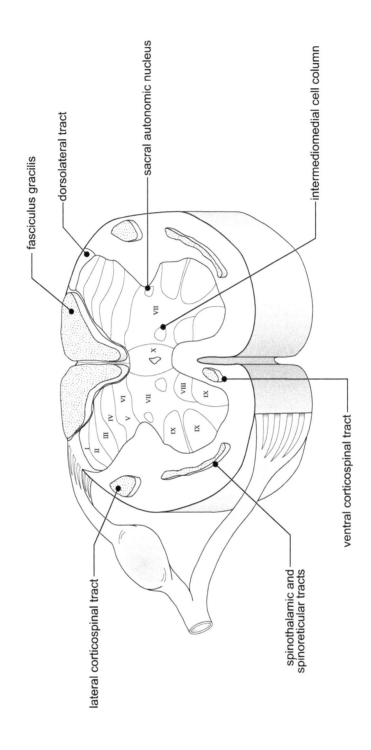

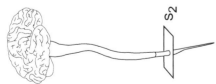

Figure 4.8   Cross section of the sacral cord

2. *Flexor reflex*: is a polysynaptic reflex. The circuitry is indicated in Figure 4.9 and summarized as follows:

Stepping on a painful stimulus stimulates nociceptors in the left foot → via Aδ and C fibers → afferent neurons in dorsal root ganglion → via dorsal root → dorsolateral tract → interneurons in dorsal gray horn → alpha motor neurons that excite flexors and inhibit extensors of the left lower limb, resulting in withdrawal of the left lower limb from a painful stimulus.

In standing or walking, interneurons also project to the contralateral alpha motor neurons to excite contralateral extensors and inhibit contralateral flexors. This is the *crossed extensor reflex*.

3. *Tendon organ reflex*: The circuitry is indicated in Figure 4.9 and summarized as follows:

Increased muscle tension → activates golgi tendon organs → via *1b* afferents → afferent neurons in dorsal root ganglion → via dorsal root → interneurons in dorsal gray horn → inhibits alpha motor neurons, resulting in decrease muscle tension

Clinical Notes:

1. *Spinal Cord Injuries*

   Monoplegia occurs with damage to the thoracic cord resulting in paralysis of one limb
   Hemiplegia occurs with a damage of the upper cervical cord resulting in paralysis of one side of the body
   Paraplegia occurs with damage between the cervical and lumbosacral enlargements of the cord and involves paralysis of both lower limbs
   Quadriplegia occurs with damage of the cervical cord and involves paralysis of the upper and lower limbs

   Spinal shock occurs immediately after a severe injury to the spinal cord. All somatic and visceral functions below the level of lesion are lost.   Several weeks after the injury, return of reflex activity occurs, tendon reflexes become hyperactive and muscles become spastic. Autonomic reflexes, such as emptying of the bowel and bladder are lost.

Brown-Sequard syndrome: incomplete transaction of the cord as a result of tumor or trauma at *T4*

- results in ipsilateral loss of discriminative touch and proprioception below the level of lesion due to lesion of the dorsal and dorsolateral funiculi of the cord
- results in contralateral loss of pain and temperature sensation below the level of lesion due to injury to the spinothalamic tract
- results in paralysis of the ipsilateral lower limb due to lesion of the lateral corticospinal tract

2. *Spinal Cord Lesions*

Upper motor neuron lesion: are lesions that affect the cerebral hemisphere, brain stem or descending tracts of the spinal cord. The symptoms associated with an upper motor neuron lesion are:
- voluntary movements are affected
- spasticity
- increased tendon reflexes
- Abnormal calcaneal tendon (plantar) reflex (Babinski sign). The *Babinski* sign, tested by stroking the sole of the foot, results in extension of the 1st toe and spreading of the other toes.

Lower motor neuron lesion: are lesions that affect the motor neurons of the ventral gray horn of the spinal cord. The symptoms associated with an lower motor neuron lesion are:
- flaccid paralysis and atrophy of muscles
- decreased muscle tone
- decreased tendon reflexes

Amyotrophic lateral sclerosis: is a progressive degenerative disorder involves degeneration of the motor system, namely the corticospinal tract; corticonuclear tract; motor nuclei of cranial nerves; motor neurons of ventral gray horn

Syringomyelia: caused by various unknown etiologies
- involves cavitation of the central canal of spinal cord that gradually extends to the peripheral parts of the cord
- pain and temperature fibers decussating in the ventral white commissure are involved, causing a decrease in pain and temperature sensations in the area of the shoulders and upper limb resulting in "yoke-like" anesthesia
- extension of the lesion results in weakness and atrophy of the muscles of the upper limb

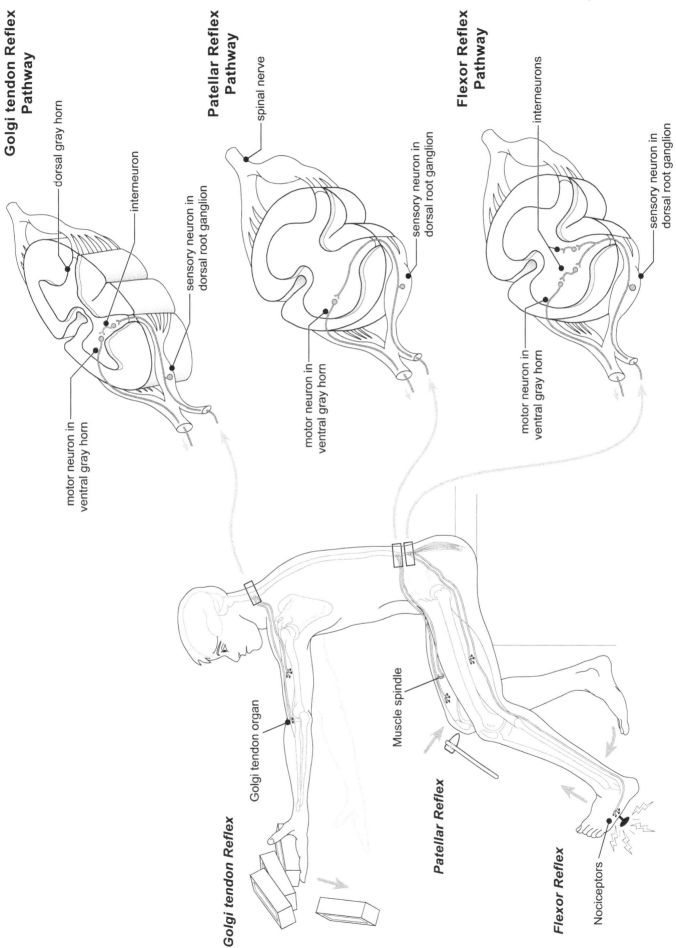

Golgi tendon Reflex Pathway

dorsal gray horn

interneuron

sensory neuron in dorsal root ganglion

motor neuron in ventral gray horn

Patellar Reflex Pathway

spinal nerve

sensory neuron in dorsal root ganglion

motor neuron in ventral gray horn

Flexor Reflex Pathway

interneurons

sensory neuron in dorsal root ganglion

motor neuron in ventral gray horn

Golgi tendon Reflex

Golgi tendon organ

Patellar Reflex

Muscle spindle

Flexor Reflex

Nociceptors

Figure 4.9   Spinal reflexes

CHAPTER
5

BRAINSTEM - EXTERNAL ANATOMY

Overview

The brainstem is superior to the spinal cord and inferior to the cerebrum. It consists of three parts, from inferior to superior are the medulla oblongata, pons and midbrain. The brainstem conducts sensory and motor tracts that convey information from the spinal cord and the cerebrum, respectively. It also consists of many motor and sensory nuclei, including autonomic and cranial nerve nuclei. Ten pairs of cranial nerves attach to the brainstem. Thus, the brainstem conducts and integrates various motor, sensory and autonomic functions.

I. Gross Anatomy of the brainstem:

A. Medulla Oblongata:

- is cone shaped and located on the occipital bone
- it lies between the pons and the spinal cord
- it consists of a **closed part** corresponding to the caudal part of the dorsal surface of the medulla. The rostral third of the dorsal surface of the medulla is the **open part**

i.   Ventral surface of medulla oblongata:

Refer to Figure 5.1 to locate the structures of the medulla oblongata

Consists of the following:

- **pyramids**, elevations on each side of the ventral median fissure and composed of corticospinal fibers
- 85% of the corticospinal fibers cross the midline in the **decussation of pyramids**, which is located at the ventral median fissure, at the junction of medulla and spinal cord
- **olive**, located lateral to the pyramid and marks the position of the **inferior olivary nucleus**
- **inferior cerebellar peduncle**, lateral to the olive and connects the medulla with the cerebellum
- rootlets of the **glossopharyngeal**, **vagus** and **accessory nerves** are attached dorsal to the olive
- the **hypoglossal nerve** emerges between the pyramid and olive

ii. Dorsal surface of medulla oblongata:

Refer to Figure 5.2 to locate the structures of the medulla oblongata

Consists of the following:

- *Open part* of medulla, located at the rostral part of medulla, and contains a portion of the *fourth* ventricle. The fourth ventricle contains cerebrospinal fluid.
- *Closed part* of the medulla narrows to the inferior end of fourth ventricle. The apex of the V-shaped inferior end of the fourth ventricle is at the *obex*, where it is continuous with the central canal of the spinal cord.
- the *fasciculus gracilis* and *fasciculus cuneatus* extends from the spinal cord, are located medially and laterally respectively, in the caudal half of the medulla
- the fasciculus gracilis and fasciculus cuneatus terminate rostrally into two swellings, the *gracile tubercle* and *cuneate tubercle*, respectively. The gracile and cuneate tubercles mark the site of the *gracile nucleus* and *cuneate nucleus*, respectively.
- the *inferior cerebellar peduncle* forms a distinct bundle of fibers on the dorsolateral border of the medulla. It consists of tracts that connect the inferior olivary nucleus, spinal cord and reticular formation with the cerebellum

B. Pons:

- is located between the medulla oblongata and the midbrain
- consists of two regions, a ventral part, referred to as the *basal* (or *basilar*) *part* and a dorsal part, referred to as the *tegmentum* of the pons

i. *Basal part:*

Refer to Figure 5.1 to locate the structures of the pons.

Consists of the following

- **basilar sulcus**, a shallow groove in the midline that contains the basilar artery
- **middle cerebellar peduncle**, located at the lateral end of the pons, is a continuation of the transverse pontine fibers (pontocerebellar fibers) that extend into the cerebellum
- the **trigeminal nerve** is located at junction of the pons and middle cerebellar peduncle
- the **abducent**, **facial** and **vestibulocochlear nerves** exit at the caudal boundary of pons, from a medial to a lateral direction, respectively

ii. *Tegmentum* or dorsal part of the pons:

Refer to Figure 5.2 to locate the structures of the pons

Consists of the following:

- rostral half of the fourth ventricle
- the *facial colliculus*, an elevation in the caudal part of the pons, in the floor of the fourth ventricle. It is formed by fibers of the facial nerve looping around the abducent nucleus
- ascending and descending tracts that originate in the forebrain, brainstem or spinal cord
- nuclear groups associated with cranial nerves
- reticular nuclei involved in sensory, motor and autonomic functions

C. Fourth Ventricle: consists of the floor, roof and lateral walls

- is located ventral to the cerebellum
- is located dorsal to the pons and rostral half of medulla

Floor of the fourth ventricle (rhomboid fossa) is divided into halves by a *median sulcus* (Figures 5.2 and 20.1) and consists of the following:

- *sulcus limitans*, divides each half of the rhomboid fossa into medial and lateral areas
- *vestibular area*, is the lateral part of rhomboid fossa and contains the *vestibular nuclear complex*
- *vagal trigone*, is located in the caudal part of the rhomboid fossa and overlies the *dorsal nucleus of vagus*
- *hypoglossal trigone*, is located in the caudal part of the rhomboid fossa and overlies the *hypoglossal nucleus*
- *medial eminence*, an elevation located at the upper half of the rhomboid fossa, medial to sulcus limitans
- *facial colliculus*, an elevation located at the lower part of the medial eminence, in the caudal pontine region, and produced by fibers of the facial nerve looping around the abducent nucleus

Roof of fourth ventricle consists of the following:

- *superior cerebellar peduncle*, forms rostral part of the roof; consists of fibers that connect the midbrain and cerebellum
- *superior medullary velum*, a thin layer of white matter located at the interval between the superior cerebellar peduncles
- *inferior medullary velum*, completes the remainder of the roof, and consists of pia mater
- *median aperture* (*foramen of Magendie*), an opening at the caudal part of the roof of fourth ventricle

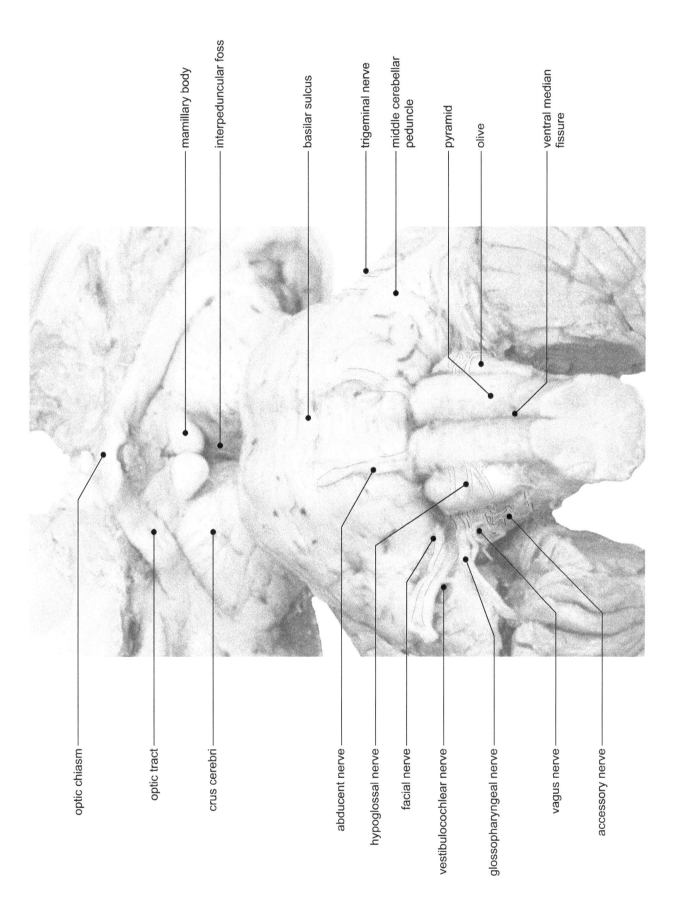

mamillary body

interpeduncular foss

basilar sulcus

trigeminal nerve

middle cerebellar peduncle

pyramid

olive

ventral median fissure

optic chiasm

optic tract

crus cerebri

abducent nerve

hypoglossal nerve

facial nerve

vestibulocochlear nerve

glossopharyngeal nerve

vagus nerve

accessory nerve

Figure 5.1   Ventral surface of the brainstem

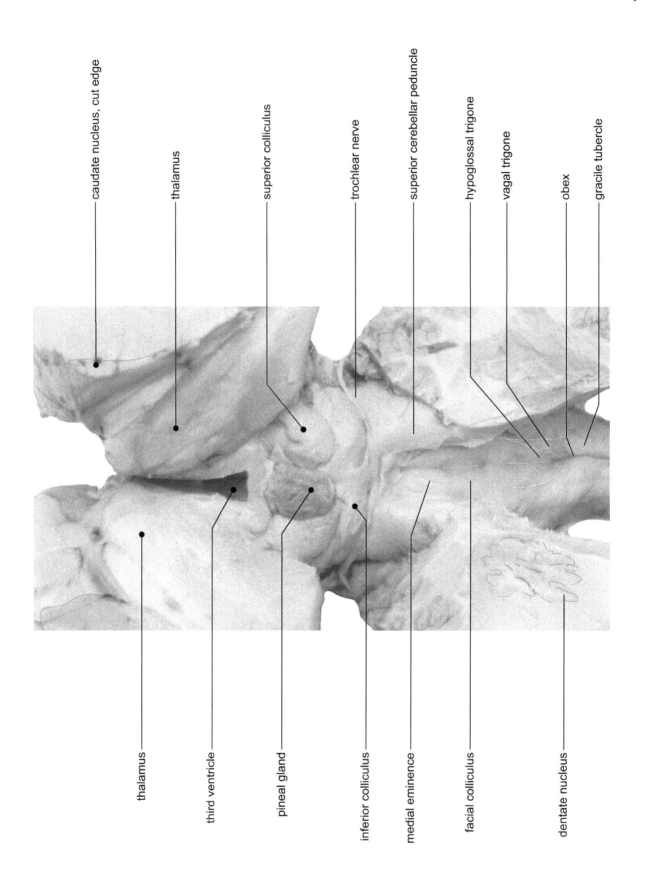

caudate nucleus, cut edge

thalamus

superior colliculus

trochlear nerve

superior cerebellar peduncle

hypoglossal trigone

vagal trigone

obex

gracile tubercle

thalamus

third ventricle

pineal gland

inferior colliculus

medial eminence

facial colliculus

dentate nucleus

Figure 5.2   Dorsal surface of the brainstem

Lateral walls of fourth ventricle consists of the following*:*

- *inferior cerebellar peduncle*, lateral to the olive; consists of fibers that connect the medulla oblongata and cerebellum
- *lateral apertures* (foramen of *Luschka*), located at the cerebellopontine angles

Cerebrospinal fluid enters the subarachnoid space through the *median aperture* and *lateral apertures*

D. Midbrain:

- extends from the pons to the mamillary bodies of the diencephalon.
- consists of two parts, the *cerebral peduncle* and *tectum*. The cerebral peduncle, in turn, includes both the *crus cerebri*, located ventrally and the *tegmentum* located dorsally
- *cerebral aqueduct,* continues with the fourth ventricle, separates the tegmentum from the tectum

Refer to Figures 5.1 and 5.2 to locate the structures of the midbrain.

i. *Ventral surface:*
- *crus cerebri* (basis pedunculi), thick bundle of descending fibers extending from the cerebrum to the brain stem and spinal cord
- *interpeduncular fossa* is located between the crus cerebri
- the *oculomotor nerve* emerges medial to the crus cerebri

ii. *Dorsal surface:*
- *corpora quadrigemina* makes up the *tectum.* Includes a pair of rounded structures, the *superior colliculi* and the *inferior colliculi*
- the *trochlear nerve* emerges below inferior colliculi and curves towards the dorsal aspect of midbrain

CHAPTER
6

BRAINSTEM - INTERNAL ORGANIZATION

Overview

The brainstem consists of many sensory and motor nuclei, including cranial nerve nuclei and the reticular formation. Motor tracts convey information from the cerebrum to the brainstem and spinal cord while sensory tracts convey information from the spinal cord to the cerebrum. Some tracts leave the brainstem while others synapse in brainstem nuclei. The internal organization of the medulla oblongata, pons and midbrain will be described in two representative sections at the caudal and rostral levels. Only important internal anatomical structures will be described. Relevant details of structures and tracts are also described in chapter 7. Details of cranial nerve nuclei and tracts will be dealt with in chapter 8.

A. Medulla Oblongata:

1. Internal Anatomy:

   a. *Caudal Medulla*:

   The following structures, traced from a dorsal to a ventral direction, in a transverse section of the caudal medulla (Figure 6.1) are:

   i. ***nucleus gracilis*** and ***fasciculus gracilis***:
      - is located medially, in the closed part of the medulla
      - conveys fine touch, proprioception, and vibration from the lower limb and lower trunk

   ii. ***nucleus cuneatus*** and ***fasciculus cuneatus:***
      - is located lateral and rostral to the nucleus gracilis
      - conveys fine touch, proprioception, and vibration from the upper trunk, arm and neck

   Efferent fibers from the nucleus gracilis and nucleus cuneatus arch ventrally as the ***internal arcuate fibers*** and cross the midline to form the contralateral ***medial lemniscus***

iii. ***external (accessory) cuneate nucleus:***
- is located lateral to the cuneate nucleus
- conveys proprioception from neck and upper limb

iv. ***spinal trigeminal nucleus***
- is located laterally
- conveys pain, temperature, light and discriminative touch from the head and face

v. ***reticular formation***:
- is located medially, and extends throughout the brainstem
- involved in regulation of motor activity, modulation of sensory input to the cortex, control of consciousness and autonomic regulation

vi. ***decussation of the pyramids:***
- located in the lower ventral part of the section (Figure 6.1)
- 85% of the corticospinal fibers cross in a dorsolateral direction to the opposite side, descending in the lateral funiculus of the spinal cord as the ***lateral corticospinal tract***. The remaining 15% of the fibers descend in the ventral funiculus of the spinal cord as the ***ventral corticospinal tract***. The corticospinal tract is involved in voluntary motor activity.

b. *Rostral Medulla*:

The following structures, traced from a dorsal to a ventral direction, in a transverse section indicated in Figure 6.1 are:

i. ***fourth ventricle***:
- is located in the upper part of the medulla and contains cerebrospinal fluid

ii. ***hypoglossal nucleus, dorsal nucleus of vagus, solitary nucleus*** and ***vestibular nuclei***
- lie from medial to lateral and located in the floor of the fourth ventricle
- the hypoglossal nucleus supplies the muscles of the tongue; the dorsal nucleus of the vagus is involved in cardiovascular control; the solitary nucleus is involved in cardiac and respiratory functions including general visceral sensation; the vestibular nuclei are involved in the control of balance

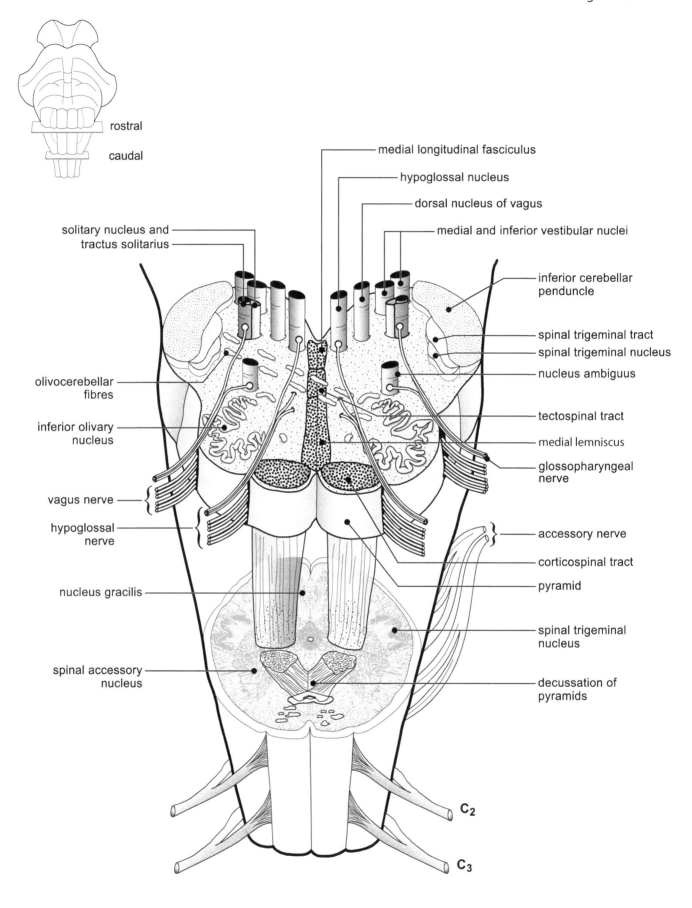

rostral

caudal

medial longitudinal fasciculus

hypoglossal nucleus

dorsal nucleus of vagus

medial and inferior vestibular nuclei

solitary nucleus and
tractus solitarius

inferior cerebellar
penduncle

spinal trigeminal tract

spinal trigeminal nucleus

nucleus ambiguus

olivocerebellar
fibres

inferior olivary
nucleus

tectospinal tract

medial lemniscus

glossopharyngeal
nerve

vagus nerve

hypoglossal
nerve

accessory nerve

corticospinal tract

nucleus gracilis

pyramid

spinal trigeminal
nucleus

spinal accessory
nucleus

decussation of
pyramids

C₂

C₃

Figure 6.1   Transverse sections of the medulla at the rostral and caudal levels

iii. *inferior cerebellar peduncle* (*restiform body*):
  - is located dorsolaterally and consists of many tracts that transmit information from the spinal cord and medulla to the cerebellum

iv. *medial lemniscus*:
  - a flattened fiber bundle located in the midline, medial to the inferior olivary nucleus
  - transmits information regarding proprioception, vibration and fine touch from the extremities to the thalamus

v. *nucleus ambiguus*:
  - is located dorsal to the inferior olivary nucleus
  - innervates muscles of the pharynx and larynx and involved in speech and swallowing

vi. *inferior olivary nucleus:*
  - located deep to the olive, shaped like a crumbled purse
  - largest nuclei of the inferior olivary complex, projects to the contralateral cerebellum via olivocerebellar fibers. It receives input from the spinal cord and the red nucleus and functions in relaying information to the cerebellum when a correction to the intended movement is required

vii. *pyramid*
  - on each side of the midline, anterior to the medial lemniscus and contains corticospinal fibers, originating from the precentral gyrus, postcentral gyrus and premotor area of the cerebral cortex

B. Pons

1. Internal Anatomy:

a. *Caudal Pons*

Refer to Figure 6.2 for structures of the caudal pons. Important structures traced from a dorsal to ventral direction are:

Tegmentum (Dorsal Pons):

i. *fourth ventricle*:
  - is located in the upper part of the pons

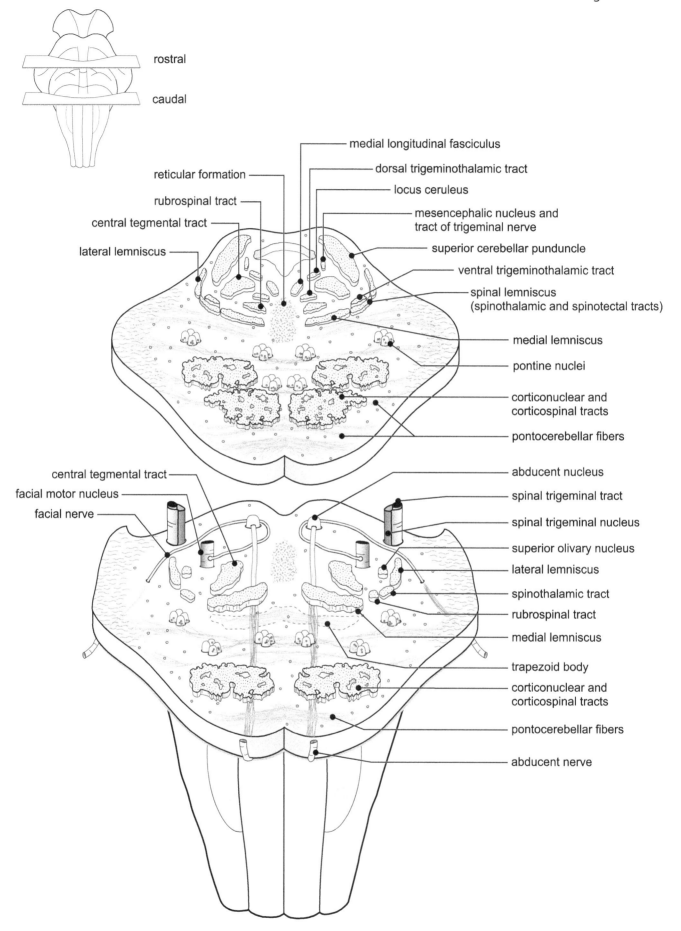

rostral

caudal

medial longitudinal fasciculus

reticular formation

dorsal trigeminothalamic tract

rubrospinal tract

locus ceruleus

central tegmental tract

mesencephalic nucleus and tract of trigeminal nerve

lateral lemniscus

superior cerebellar punduncle

ventral trigeminothalamic tract

spinal lemniscus (spinothalamic and spinotectal tracts)

medial lemniscus

pontine nuclei

corticonuclear and corticospinal tracts

pontocerebellar fibers

central tegmental tract

abducent nucleus

facial motor nucleus

spinal trigeminal tract

facial nerve

spinal trigeminal nucleus

superior olivary nucleus

lateral lemniscus

spinothalamic tract

rubrospinal tract

medial lemniscus

trapezoid body

corticonuclear and corticospinal tracts

pontocerebellar fibers

abducent nerve

Figure 6.2   Transverse sections of the pons at the rostral and caudal levels

    ii. *middle cerebellar peduncle*
- located laterally, contains transverse fibers that connect the pons with the cerebellum

    iii. *abducent nucleus*:
- located in the floor of the fourth ventricle
- supplies the lateral rectus muscle, which abducts the eye

    iv. *facial nucleus*:
- lies in the ventrolateral aspect, where fibers run dorsomedially and course over the abducent nucleus, forming the *facial colliculus*. Fibers of the facial nerve continue ventrolaterally, exits at the lower border of the pons, and innervates ipsilateral facial muscles

Ventral or Basal Pons

    i. ***corticospinal and corticonuclear fibers*** become dispersed in the basal pons as longitudinal bundles of fibers, among the transverse pontine fibers.

    ii. ***pontine nuclei*** are interspersed among the transverse pontine fibers and receive input from the ipsilateral cerebral cortex (corticopontine fibers). The axons of the pontine nuclei form the transverse pontine fibers (***pontocerebellar fibers***)

    iii. ***pontocerebellar fibers*** are postsynaptic axons of pontine nuclei that cross the midline and enter the contralateral cerebellum via the middle cerebellar peduncle. This projection forms a major pathway by which the cerebral cortex (corticopontine fibers) communicates with the cerebellar cortex (***pontocerebellar fibers***).

b. *Rostral Pons*

Refer to Figure 6.2 for structures of the rostral pons. Important structures traced from a dorsal to ventral direction are:

Tegmentum (Dorsal Pons):

    i. ***fourth ventricle***
- is located in the upper part of the pons and narrows as it becomes continuous with the cerebral aqueduct

    ii. ***superior cerebellar peduncle*** forms the roof of the fourth ventricle
- contains efferents to the midbrain and thalamus
- at the rostral border of the pons, the superior cerebellar peduncles are joined by the ***superior medullary velum***, which forms the roof of the fourth ventricle

Ventral or Basal Pons

  i. ***corticospinal and corticonuclear fibers*** become dispersed in the basal pons. Many corticonuclear fibers terminate in motor nuclei of cranial nerves
  ii. ***pontine nuclei*** are interspersed among the transverse pontine fibers
  iii. ***pontocerebellar fibers*** cross the midline and enter the middle cerebellar peduncle

C. Midbrain

1. Internal Anatomy:

The midbrain consists of the *tectum*, *tegmentum* and *basis pedunculi* (crus cerebri).

 a. <u>*Level of the Inferior Colliculus*</u>

  Refer to Figure 6.3 for structures of the midbrain. Important structures traced from a dorsal to ventral direction are:

  Tectum : region of the midbrain dorsal to cerebral aqueduct and consists of four elevations, the ***corpora quadrigemina***. The corpora quadrigemina consists of a pair of superior colliculi and inferior colliculi

   i. ***inferior colliculi:***
    • is a component of the auditory pathway and also regulates auditory reflexes

   ii. ***cerebral aqueduct***:
    • narrow canal that connects the third ventricle with the fourth ventricle and contains cerebrospinal fluid

  Tegmentum:

   iii. ***periaqueductal gray***:
    • gray matter around the cerebral aqueduct
    • consists of neurons that project to the **nucleus raphe magnus** of the medulla, a pathway that plays a significant role in suppression of pain

   iv. ***reticular formation***:
    • consists of many nuclei and fiber tracts

   v. ***decussation of the superior cerebellar peduncle:***
    • is located in the central area of the tegmentum, ventral to the cerebral aqueduct

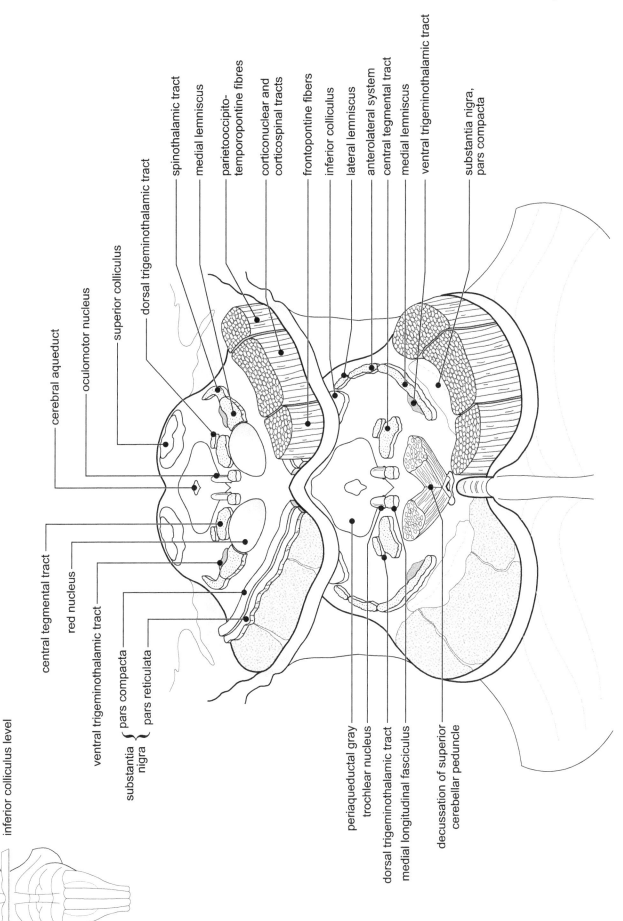

Figure 6.3   Transverse sections of the midbrain at the levels of the superior and inferior colliculi

superior colliculus level

inferior colliculus level

spinothalamic tract

medial lemniscus

parietooccipito-temporopontine fibres

corticonuclear and corticospinal tracts

frontopontine fibers

inferior colliculus

lateral lemniscus

anterolateral system

central tegmental tract

medial lemniscus

ventral trigeminothalamic tract

substantia nigra, pars compacta

cerebral aqueduct

oculomotor nucleus

superior colliculus

dorsal trigeminothalamic tract

central tegmental tract

red nucleus

ventral trigeminothalamic tract

substantia nigra { pars compacta / pars reticulata }

periaqueductal gray

trochlear nucleus

dorsal trigeminothalamic tract

medial longitudinal fasciculus

decussation of superior cerebellar peduncle

- includes fibers that cross the midline as they ascend to the red nucleus and thalamus

Substantia nigra:
- is located between the tegmentum and the basis pedunculi
- extends into the subthalamic region of diencephalon
- is part of the basal ganglia
- consists of two parts, the ***pars compacta*** and ***pars reticulata***. Neurons of the ***pars compacta***, located adjacent to the tegmentum, contain granules of ***neuromelanin***, a byproduct of dopamine metabolism. These neurons project to the striatum and modulate the level of activity of the striatal neurons in both the direct and indirect circuits of the basal ganglia. Neurons of the ***pars reticulata***, located dorsal to the basis pedunculi, do not contain neuromelanin. It is considered to be similar to the GABA-ergic neurons of the internal segment of the globus pallidus. The substantia nigra has a regulatory effect on the corpus striatum, regulates muscle tone and motor coordination

Clinical Notes:

Degeneration of neurons of the pars compacta leads to decrease in dopamine, resulting in ***Parkinson's disease***. Clinical features are muscular rigidity, resting tremor and difficulty in initiating movements. Parkinson's disease is treated with ***levodopa***, a precursor of dopamine that can be transported through the blood-brain barrier. Other treatments such as transplantation of fetal dopamine-producing tissue, surgical ablation of the medial pallidum or implantation of electrodes in the thalamus have had some success in treating advanced cases of Parkinson's disease

Crus cerebri (basis pedunculi):
- consists of tracts that arise from the cerebral cortex, which terminate within the brainstem (corticonuclear fibers) or within the spinal cord (corticospinal fibers). The crus cerebri is organized as follows:
  - a. fibers in the medial fifth contain *frontopontine fibers* that terminate in the pontine nuclei
  - b. fibers in the middle three-fifths constitute the corticospinal and corticonuclear (corticobulbar) fibers
  - c. fibers in the lateral fifth contain parietotemporopontine fibers (including fibers from the occipital lobe) that terminate in the pontine nuclei

b. _Level of the Superior Colliculus_

Refer to Figure 6.3 for structures of the midbrain. Important structures traced from a dorsal to ventral direction are:

Tectum:

    i. **superior colliculi:**
        • is a component of the visual pathway and also regulates visual reflexes
        • also projects to the cervical cord via the _tectospinal tract_ for reflex movements of the head and neck in response to sensory input

    ii. **cerebral aqueduct**:
        • narrow canal that connects the third ventricle with the fourth ventricle

Tegmentum:

    iii. **periaqueductal gray**:
        • gray matter around the cerebral aqueduct that plays an important role in suppression of pain

    iv. **reticular formation**:
        • consists of many nuclei and fiber tracts

    v. **red nucleus:**
        • round nucleus, located in the central area of the tegmentum
        • extends from the level of the superior colliculus into the subthalamic region of the diencephalon
        • it receives information from the cerebral cortex and cerebellum and projects to the spinal cord, cerebellum and inferior olivary nucleus. The red nucleus functions in control of flexor muscles of the arm

    Substantia nigra:
        • is located between the tegmentum and the basis pedunculi (described above)

    Crus cerebri (basis pedunculi): consists of tracts that arise from the cerebral cortex that terminate within the brainstem (corticonuclear fibers) or within the spinal cord (corticospinal fibers).

Clinical Notes:

Brainstem lesions occur mainly as a result of vascular disorders. Vascular lesions can involve the lateral, medial, ventral or dorsal areas of the brainstem. Different combinations of neurological deficits will depend on the size and location of the area affected. A single lesion of the brainstem commonly involves many structures since many sensory and motor tracts, nuclei of cranial nerves (Chapter 8) and reticular nuclei (Chapter 9) are located in the brainstem. Location and neurological deficits of more common lesions in the medulla, pons and midbrain are described below.

Medulla:
Lateral Medullary (or *Wallenburg*) *Syndrome* results from a vascular lesion of the vertebral and the posterior inferior cerebellar arteries. This syndrome involves loss of pain and temperature from the ipsilateral face; loss of the gag reflex and difficulty in swallowing and speech; dizziness and ataxia; constriction of the pupil and drooping of the upper eyelid (*Horner's syndrome*). Structures affected include the spinothalamic tract; spinal trigeminal nucleus and tract; nucleus ambiguus; vestibular nuclei and descending autonomic fibers from the forebrain and brainstem. *Medial Medullary Syndrome* results from a vascular lesion of the anterior spinal artery or branches of the vertebral artery. This syndrome involves loss of proprioception, touch and pressure from the contralateral side of the body; contralateral paralysis, paralysis of the ipsilateral tongue and ipsilateral deviation of the tongue upon protrusion. Structures affected include the corticospinal tract, medial lemniscus and rootlets of the hypoglossal nerve.

Pons:
Raymond's Syndrome results from a lesion of the pontine branches of the basilar artery that supplies the caudal basal aspect of the pons. This syndrome involves contralateral hemiplegia and medial strabismus of the ipsilateral eye. Structures affected include the corticospinal tract as well as the abducent nerve if the lesion extends far enough medially. *Foville's Syndrome* results from a lesion of the branches of the basilar artery that supplies the dorsal and medial aspects of the pons. This syndrome involves ipsilateral facial paralysis and lateral gaze paralysis in combination with internuclear ophthalmoplegia. Structures affected include the facial nerve together with the abducent nucleus, the paramedian pontine reticular formation and the medial longitudinal fasciculus.

Midbrain:
Weber's Syndrome results from a lesion of the branches of the posterior cerebral artery. This syndrome involves ipsilateral oculomotor nerve palsy and contralateral hemiplegia with paralysis of the lower part of the face, tongue including the arm and leg. Oculomotor nerve involvement includes lateral strabismus, ptosis and dilation of the pupil. Structures affected include the rootlets of the oculomotor nerve and the medial part of the crus cerebri. *Benedikt's Syndrome* is similar to Weber's syndrome, but the lesion extends further dorsally to include regions of the red nucleus, superior cerebellar peduncle and adjoining parts of the medial lemniscus and spinothalamic tract. This syndrome involves ipsilateral oculomotor nerve palsy, contralateral somatosensory loss, as well as tremor of the opposite limb.

CHAPTER
7

SOMATOSENSORY AND MOTOR TRACTS

Overview

Sensory systems include somatic and special senses. Special senses include vision, auditory, vestibular, taste and olfaction. Motor systems include all descending pathways that influence motor activity. These pathways arise from the cerebral cortex to terminate in the brainstem or the spinal cord. In addition, subcortical nuclei influence motor activity via feedback circuits that link the cerebral cortex, basal ganglia, cerebellum and spinal cord. Knowledge of the location and functions of nuclei and tracts will help in understanding various motor and sensory deficits in brain injuries.

I. Somatosensory Pathways:

Somatic sensations are conveyed to the primary sensory cortex via an organization of three neurons. The *first-order neurons*, in the dorsal root ganglion, convey sensory information from the periphery and transmit it to *second-order neurons* in the spinal cord or the brainstem. Axons of second-order neurons cross the midline, ascend to the opposite side and relay in the thalamus, which contain *third-order neurons.* Third-order neurons project to the cerebral cortex.

The somatosensory system can be divided into the *dorsomedial system* (*medial lemniscus system* or *posterior column system*); pathways to the cerebellum and the *anterolateral system*. The *trigeminothalamic pathway* for the head will be described with the description of the cranial nerves. The medial lemniscus system conveys discriminative touch, vibration, proprioception and deep pressure; cerebellar pathways convey conscious and unconscious proprioception. The anterolateral system conveys pain, temperature and light touch

A. Medial Lemniscus (Figure 7.1)– conveys discriminative or fine touch; proprioception, vibration from the upper limbs, trunk and lower limbs

- Information from sensory receptors via 1a; Aβ fibers to:

    ⇒ dorsal root ganglia, containing cell bodies of sensory neurons
    ⇒ via medial division of dorsal roots

⇒ *fasciculus gracilis* (caudal to T6, from the lumbar and lower thoracic nerves) synapsing in *nucleus gracilis*

or to

⇒ *fasciculus cuneatus* (rostral to T6, from the upper thoracic and cervical nerves) synapsing in *nucleus cuneatus*

⇒ axons curve ventrally as the *internal arcuate fibers*

⇒ cross the midline in the *decussation of the medial lemniscus*

⇒ ascends in the tegmentum of the pons and midbrain

⇒ synapses in the ventral posterior lateral nucleus of the thalamus

⇒ via the posterior limb of internal capsule

⇒ to the primary sensory area of the cerebral cortex

The integrity of the medial lemniscus system is tested by the following: joint position sense, vibratory sense and two-point discrimination tests.

The *Romberg test* is used to evaluate proprioception. The subject stands with feet together, eyes closed. Unsteadiness indicates decrease proprioception from the lower limbs.

B. Pathways to the Cerebellum:

Spinocerebellar tracts: convey proprioception from lower limbs

i.   *Dorsal spinocerebellar tract* (Figure 7.2) - conveys proprioception from the lower limbs

• Information from muscle spindles:

⇒ via lumbar and sacral dorsal nerve roots (medial division)

⇒ synapse in *nucleus thoracicus* (*nucleus dorsalis*)

⇒ axons ascend ipsilaterally as *dorsal spinocerebellar tract*

⇒ ascends through the dorsolateral funiculus of the spinal cord

⇒ ipsilateral inferior cerebellar peduncle

⇒ terminates in the cerebellar cortex

ii.   *Ventral spinocerebellar tract* (Figure 7.2) - conveys proprioception from lower limbs

• Information from golgi tendon organs:

⇒ dorsal root ganglia

⇒ via lumbar and sacral dorsal nerve roots

⇒ synapse in the lumbosacral enlargement of cord

⇒ fibers cross in ventral white commissure

⇒ ascends in the dorsolateral funiculus of spinal cord

⇒ ascends in the tegmentum of the medulla and pons

⇒ joins the superior cerebellar peduncle

⇒ fibers cross to the contralateral side

⇒ terminates in the cerebellar cortex

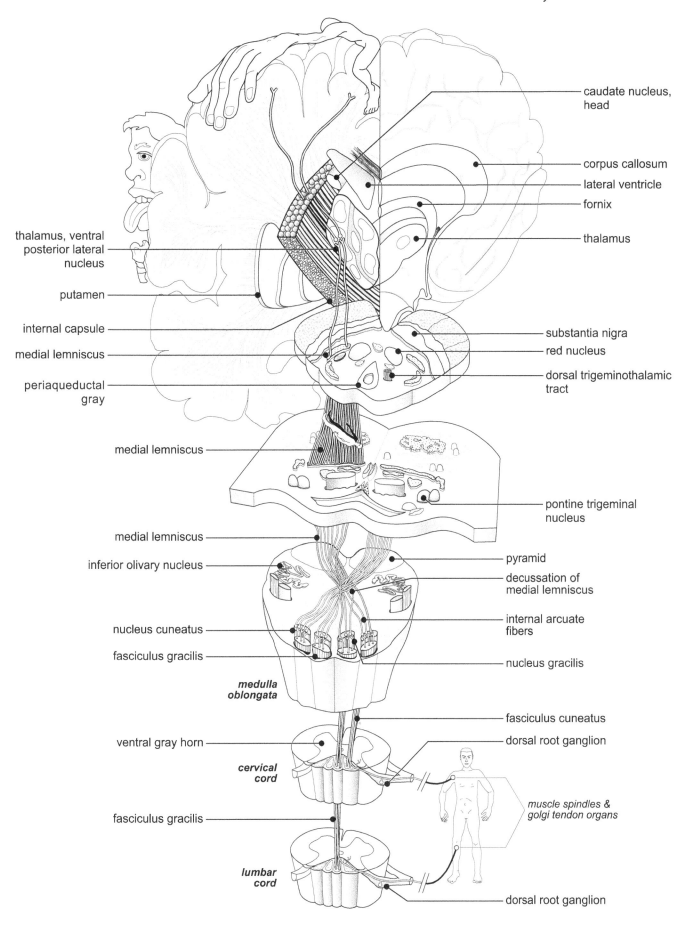

caudate nucleus, head

corpus callosum

lateral ventricle

fornix

thalamus

thalamus, ventral posterior lateral nucleus

putamen

internal capsule

medial lemniscus

periaqueductal gray

substantia nigra

red nucleus

dorsal trigeminothalamic tract

medial lemniscus

pontine trigeminal nucleus

medial lemniscus

inferior olivary nucleus

pyramid

decussation of medial lemniscus

internal arcuate fibers

nucleus cuneatus

fasciculus gracilis

nucleus gracilis

medulla oblongata

fasciculus cuneatus

ventral gray horn

dorsal root ganglion

cervical cord

muscle spindles & golgi tendon organs

fasciculus gracilis

lumbar cord

dorsal root ganglion

Figure 7.1   Medial lemniscus system

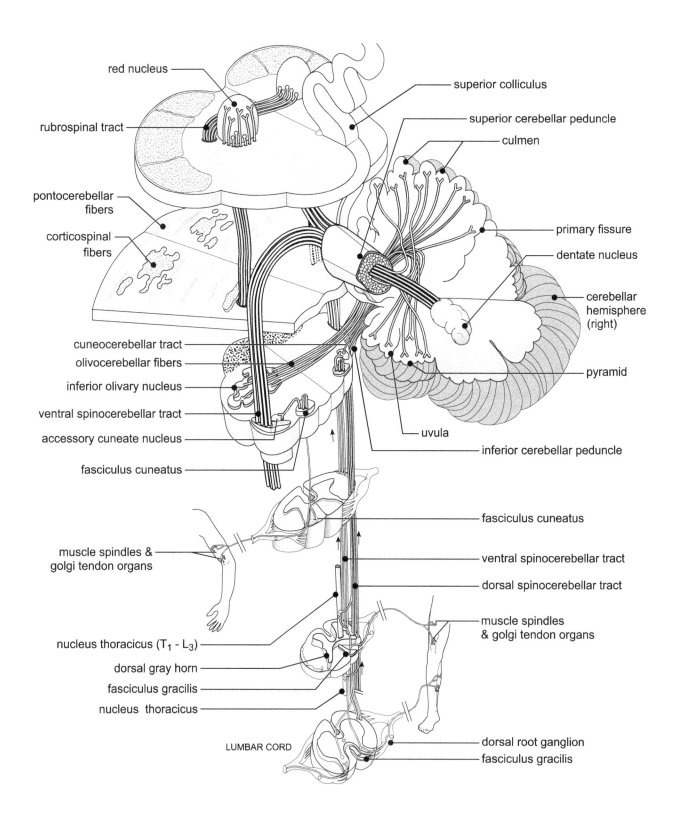

red nucleus

rubrospinal tract

pontocerebellar fibers

corticospinal fibers

cuneocerebellar tract

olivocerebellar fibers

inferior olivary nucleus

ventral spinocerebellar tract

accessory cuneate nucleus

fasciculus cuneatus

muscle spindles & golgi tendon organs

nucleus thoracicus (T$_1$ - L$_3$)

dorsal gray horn

fasciculus gracilis

nucleus thoracicus

LUMBAR CORD

superior colliculus

superior cerebellar peduncle

culmen

primary fissure

dentate nucleus

cerebellar hemisphere (right)

pyramid

uvula

inferior cerebellar peduncle

fasciculus cuneatus

ventral spinocerebellar tract

dorsal spinocerebellar tract

muscle spindles & golgi tendon organs

dorsal root ganglion

fasciculus gracilis

Figure 7.2   Dorsal and ventral spinocerebellar tracts and olivocerebellar tract

iii. ***Cuneocerebellar tract*** (Figure 7.2) - conveys proprioception from upper limb

- Information from muscle spindles:

  ⇒ dorsal root ganglia
  ⇒ via cervical dorsal nerve roots
  ⇒ dorsal funiculus of spinal cord
  ⇒ ascends in the fasciculus cuneatus
  ⇒ collaterals from fasciculus cuneatus synapse in ***accessory cuneate nucleus***
  ⇒ ascends in the ipsilateral inferior cerebellar peduncle
  ⇒ terminates in the cerebellum (vermis and paravermal area)

C. Anterolateral system: is involved in conveying pain, temperature and light touch. It includes the ***spinothalamic, spinomesencephalic (spinotectal)*** and ***spinoreticular*** pathways

The first type of pain is felt as sharp and localized. It is referred to as ***fast pain*** and is of short duration. This type of pain is conducted by myelinated group Aδ fibers. The second type of pain is called ***slow pain***. It is diffuse and poorly localized and is chronic pain. This type of pain is conducted by unmyelinated group C fibers. A third type of pain arises from internal organs and is called ***referred pain***. Referred pain is poorly localized and is commonly referred to an area of the body surface. Pain from visceral nociceptors (result of peritonitis, ischemia) causes pain perception as somatic and corresponds to a dermatome innervated by the spinal segment to which visceral afferents project. Visceral and somatic afferents converge onto the ventral posterior lateral nucleus of the thalamus.

Examples are:
i. heart: T1 to T5 spinal segments
ii. appendix - T10 spinal segment
iii. ureter, kidney - L1 to L2 spinal segments

Spinothalamic tract (Figure 7.3) - conveys pain, temperature, light touch

- Pain from nociceptors via Aδ and C fibers to:

  ⇒ dorsal root ganglion
  ⇒ dorsal root (lateral division)
  ⇒ dorsolateral tract of Lissauer
  ⇒ fibers ascend or descend a few spinal segments
  ⇒ synapse in lamina I and II, axons of these neurons synapse in laminae 1V-V1 (tract cells)
  ⇒ axons of tract cells cross in the anterior white commissure to the contralateral side to form the ***spinothalamic tract***
  ⇒ in the lateral funiculus of the spinal cord

⇒ ascend in the medulla, tegmentum of pons and midbrain

⇒ synapse in ventral posterior lateral nucleus of thalamus

⇒ via the posterior limb of internal capsule

⇒ to terminate in the primary sensory area of the cerebral cortex

Clinical Notes:

Injury to the spinothalamic tract in the spinal cord or brainstem would result in contralateral loss of pain and temperature below the level of lesion. Surgical interruption (*cordotomy* or *tractotomy*) of the spinothalamic tract at the level of the spinal cord is sometimes employed to eliminate intractable pain.

II. Motor Systems:

Descending tracts are classified as controlling skilled voluntary movements (***corticospinal*** and ***corticonuclear tracts***) or those that are involved in maintaining posture and coordination of movement (***basal ganglia***, ***cerebellum***).

A. Major descending pathways

1. Corticospinal tract (Figure 7.4)

- Fibers arise from the premotor, primary motor area, primary sensory area and supplementary motor area of the cortex

    ⇒ travel via the posterior limb of the internal capsule

    ⇒ through the middle 3/5 of the basis pedunculi, from medial to lateral are fibers for the neck, arm, trunk and leg

    ⇒ descends through the basilar pons, breaks up into fasciculi between bundles of corticopontine fibers

    ⇒ corticospinal fibers (pyramidal tract) descend through the ventral surface of the medulla, referred to as the ***pyramid***

    ⇒ 85 % of fibers cross the midline at the junction of the medulla and the spinal cord, in the ***decussation of the pyramid***

    ⇒ enter the lateral funiculus of the spinal cord as the ***lateral corticospinal tract***

    ⇒ the remaining 15% of the fibers descend in the ventral funiculus as the ***ventral corticospinal tract***, and decussate at segmental levels of the cord

    ⇒ most fibers terminate in laminae 1V - V11; 1X of the spinal cord

    function: controls skilled voluntary movements of the extremities (lateral corticospinal tract); supply axial musculature (ventral corticospinal tract)

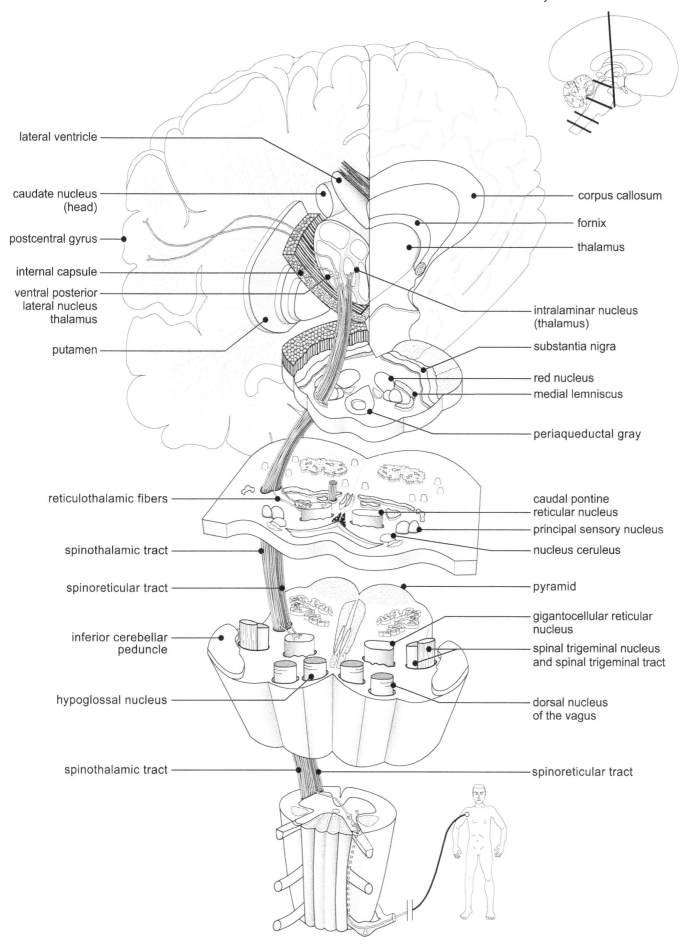

lateral ventricle

caudate nucleus
(head)

postcentral gyrus

internal capsule

ventral posterior
lateral nucleus
thalamus

putamen

corpus callosum

fornix

thalamus

intralaminar nucleus
(thalamus)

substantia nigra

red nucleus

medial lemniscus

periaqueductal gray

reticulothalamic fibers

spinothalamic tract

spinoreticular tract

inferior cerebellar
peduncle

hypoglossal nucleus

spinothalamic tract

caudal pontine
reticular nucleus

principal sensory nucleus

nucleus ceruleus

pyramid

gigantocellular reticular
nucleus

spinal trigeminal nucleus
and spinal trigeminal tract

dorsal nucleus
of the vagus

spinoreticular tract

Figure 7.3   Spinothalamic and spinoreticular tracts

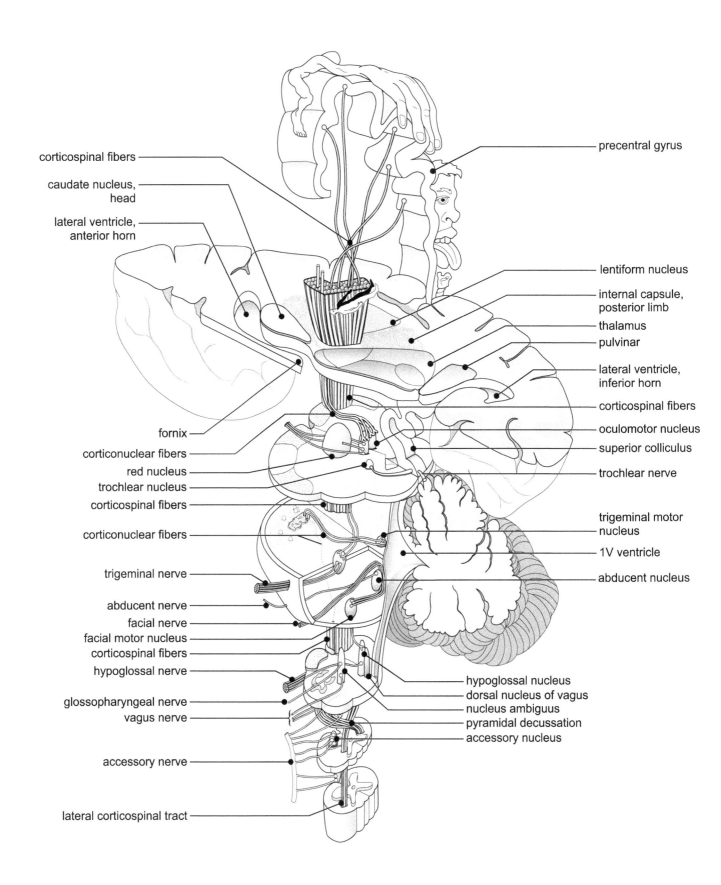

corticospinal fibers

caudate nucleus,
head

lateral ventricle,
anterior horn

precentral gyrus

lentiform nucleus

internal capsule,
posterior limb

thalamus

pulvinar

lateral ventricle,
inferior horn

corticospinal fibers

oculomotor nucleus

superior colliculus

trochlear nerve

fornix

corticonuclear fibers

red nucleus

trochlear nucleus

corticospinal fibers

corticonuclear fibers

trigeminal motor
nucleus

1V ventricle

abducent nucleus

trigeminal nerve

abducent nerve

facial nerve

facial motor nucleus

corticospinal fibers

hypoglossal nerve

glossopharyngeal nerve

vagus nerve

hypoglossal nucleus

dorsal nucleus of vagus

nucleus ambiguus

pyramidal decussation

accessory nucleus

accessory nerve

lateral corticospinal tract

Figure 7.4   Corticospinal and corticonuclear tracts

Clinical Notes:
Injury to the corticospinal tract results in paralysis of muscles; increased muscle tone; abnormal stretch reflexes and *Babinski* sign. If the lesion is above the level of the pyramidal decussation, the paralysis is contralateral to the site of lesion. If the lesion is below the pyramidal decussation, the paralysis is ipsilateral to the site of lesion.

2. Corticonuclear (corticobulbar) tract (Figure 7.4)

- originates in the motor cortex
- is located medial to the corticospinal tract, travels through the posterior limb of the internal capsule
- terminates on cranial nerve nuclei
- most terminate bilaterally

B. Other Descending Pathways

Includes the ***rubrospinal, tectospinal, reticulospinal, vestibulospinal tracts***. The latter two tracts will be described in Chapters 9 and 19

1. Rubrospinal Tract (Figure 10.7):

Afferents:
- from deep cerebellar nuclei (cerebellorubral fibers) and from premotor and motor cortex (corticorubral fibers)

Efferents:
i. rubrospinal fibers cross, descend through the tegmentum of the brainstem, descend through the lateral funiculus of the spinal cord, anterior to the corticospinal tract. The ***rubrospinal tract*** is a rudimentary tract in the human brain and its fibers terminate in the upper cervical segments of the spinal cord, synapsing with interneurons that influence motor neurons that innervate flexors of the upper limb

ii. to ipsilateral inferior olivary nucleus via the ***central tegmental tract***. In turn, the inferior olivary nucleus projects to the cerebellum

function: the red nucleus facilitates motor neurons to flexors and inhibits motor neurons to extensors

2.   *Tectospinal Tract:*

Afferents:
- corticotectal fibers from visual cortex, visual association cortex and frontal eye field to the superior colliculus

Efferents:
- tectospinal fibers cross, travel through the tegmentum of the brainstem, and descend through the ventral funiculus of the spinal cord, close to the ventral median fissure. The tectospinal tract terminates in the cervical and upper thoracic segments of the cord

function: concerned with postural movements in response to visual stimuli

CHAPTER
8

CRANIAL NERVES

Overview

Cranial nerves are peripheral nerves that arise from the brain. There are twelve pairs of cranial nerves that innervate the structures of the head and neck including the thoracic and abdominal viscera. Cranial nerves I and II arise from the forebrain, the remaining ten nerves arise from the brainstem. Cranial nerves are either sensory or motor and some nerves have both sensory and motor functions or parasympathetic functions. Cell bodies of sensory neurons of cranial nerves are generally located in ganglia outside the central nervous system. Motor neurons are located in specific nuclei in the brainstem. Motor neurons innervating muscles of the head and neck are classified as lower motor neurons.

I. General Location:

- located from anterior to posterior on the ventral surface of the brain (Figure 5.1) are the following nerves:

   Olfactory; *Optic*; *Oculomotor*; *Trochlear*; *Trigeminal*; *Abducent*, *Facial*;
   Vestibulocochlear; *Glossopharyngeal*; *Vagus*; *Accessory* and *Hypoglossal*
   (Figure 13.3)

II. Functional components of cranial nerves:

- *general somatic efferents*: supply muscles of the eye (III, IV,VI) and tongue (XII)
- *general somatic afferents*: convey various sensations of touch, pain, temperature and proprioception from skin and muscles of the head, neck and face (V,VII,IX,X)
- *special somatic afferents*: convey special senses eg. vision (II), hearing and balance (VIII)
- *general visceral afferents*: convey general sensations from visceral organs (IX,X)
- *special visceral afferents*: conveys smell (I) and taste (VII,IX,X)
- *general visceral efferents*: supply smooth muscle and glands (III,VII,IX,X) via the autonomic nervous system

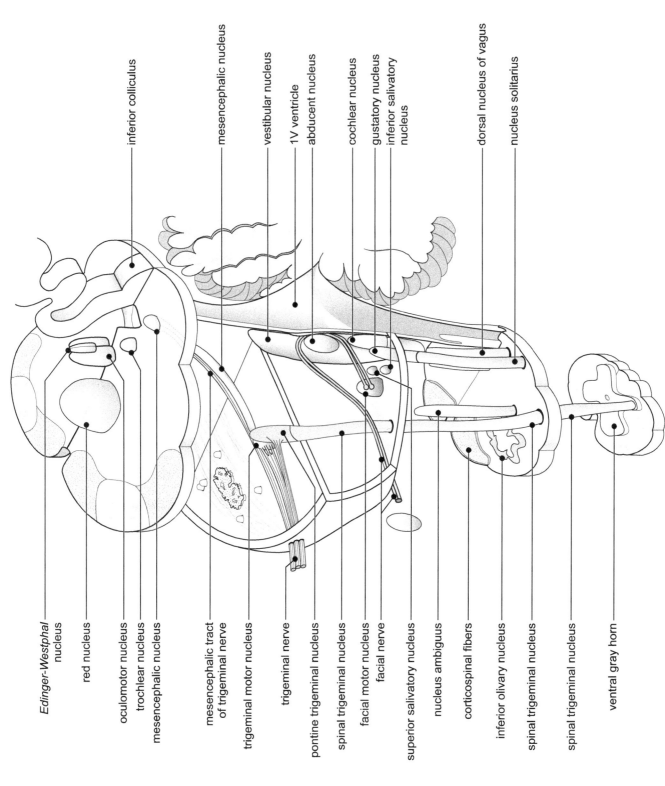

inferior colliculus

mesencephalic nucleus

vestibular nucleus

1V ventricle

abducent nucleus

cochlear nucleus

gustatory nucleus

inferior salivatory nucleus

dorsal nucleus of vagus

nucleus solitarius

Edinger-Westphal nucleus

red nucleus

oculomotor nucleus

trochlear nucleus

mesencephalic nucleus

mesencephalic tract of trigeminal nerve

trigeminal motor nucleus

trigeminal nerve

pontine trigeminal nucleus

spinal trigeminal nucleus

facial motor nucleus

facial nerve

superior salivatory nucleus

nucleus ambiguus

corticospinal fibers

inferior olivary nucleus

spinal trigeminal nucleus

spinal trigeminal nucleus

ventral gray horn

Figure 8.1   Arrangement of cranial nerve nuclei in the brainstem

III. Origin, Distribution and Functions of Cranial Nerves:

The *Olfactory*, *Optic* and *Vestibulocochlear* nerves will be described in Chapters 16, 18 and 19 respectively

A. Oculomotor, Trochlear, Abducent Nerves

The oculomotor, trochlear and abducent nerves are motor, innervating the extraocular muscles. (Figures 8.2, 8.3 and 8.4, 13.3).

The nuclei of the three nerves are interconnected to track moving objects in the visual field. In addition, the oculomotor nerve controls reflex constriction of the pupil.

1. Nuclei:

a. ***oculomotor nuclear complex:***
   - is located at level of superior colliculus of midbrain (Figure 8.1). It supplies the following five muscles that insert on the external surface of the eyeball (Figures 8.2 to 8.4). These are:
       - ***inferior rectus***: depresses the eye and rotates it medially
       - ***medial rectus***: adducts the eye
       - ***inferior oblique***: elevates the eye and rotates eye outward
       - ***superior rectus***: elevates eye and rotates it medially
       - ***levator palpebrae superioris***: elevates upper eyelid

b. ***Edinger-Westphal nucleus:***
   - is the parasympathetic nucleus and lies dorsal to the oculomotor nucleus (Figure 8.1).
   - it supplies the ***sphincter pupillae*** muscle of iris and the ***ciliary*** muscle

c. ***trochlear nucleus***
   - is located at level of inferior colliculus of midbrain (Figure 8.1).
   - it supplies the ***superior oblique***, which depresses and outwardly rotates the eye

d. ***abducent nucleus***
   - is located in the pontine tegmentum, at the level of the facial colliculus
   - it supplies the ***lateral rectus***, which abducts the eye

2. Control of eye movements:

The following muscles act together to control eye movements. Examples are:
- superior rectus and inferior oblique - elevates eye
- inferior rectus and superior oblique - depresses eye
- medial recti - adducts eye
- lateral rectus (right) and medial rectus (left) – abducts the eye (right eye)

Clinical Notes:
- lesion of the oculomotor nerve (Figure 8.5) results in ***ptosis*** (drooping of the eyelid); ***lateral strabismus*** (due to unopposed lateral rectus); dilated ***pupil*** due to loss of accommodation and ***diplopia*** (double vision)
- lesion of the trochlear nerve results in diplopia on looking down, for example, when descending stairs
- lesion of the abducent nerve (Figure 8.6) results in ***medial strabismus*** (due to unopposed medial rectus)

3. Coordinated movements of both eyes (conjugate movements)

Coordinated eye movements are controlled by the cerebral cortex. These movements are:

a. ***Smooth pursuit movements:***
  - are slow movements that are involuntary
  - is controlled by the ***posterior parietal eye field***

b. ***Voluntary eye movements*** (*conjugate lateral gaze*):
  - are rapid movements that are voluntary eg. reading a printed page
  - is controlled by the ***frontal eye field***, which stimulates gaze to the contralateral side

For example, looking to the left results in contraction of the left lateral rectus and right medial rectus. The pathway is as follows:

- from the ***right frontal eye field*** via corticotectal fibers to:
  - $\Rightarrow$ right superior colliculus
  - $\Rightarrow$ descends through cerebral peduncle
  - $\Rightarrow$ fibers cross in the pons, descend in the **medial longitudinal fasciculus**
  - $\Rightarrow$ synapse in ***paramedian pontine reticular formation*** (left)
  - $\Rightarrow$ axons synapse in abducent nucleus (left) and fibers supply the left lateral rectus
  - $\Rightarrow$ axons from the abducent nucleus exit, cross and ascend in the contralateral medial longitudinal fasciculus (Figure 10.5)
  - $\Rightarrow$ terminates in the oculomotor nucleus (right), which supplies the right medial rectus

Clinical Notes:
a. lesion of the *frontal eye field* affects lateral gaze to the contralateral side and the eye deviates to the side of the lesion
b. ***Internuclear ophthalmoplegia*** eg. in multiple sclerosis
  - lesion of the medial longitudinal fasciculus, in the rostral pons, results in the inability to adduct the ipsilateral eye due to interruption of the connections from the contralateral abducent nucleus to the ipsilateral oculomotor nucleus.

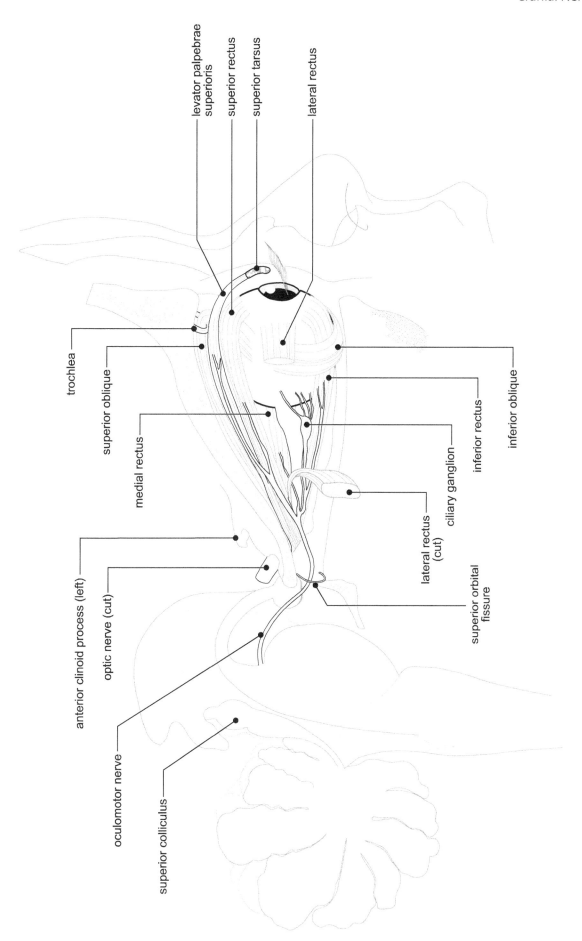

levator palpebrae superioris

superior rectus

superior tarsus

lateral rectus

trochlea

superior oblique

medial rectus

anterior clinoid process (left)

optic nerve (cut)

oculomotor nerve

superior colliculus

inferior oblique

inferior rectus

ciliary ganglion

lateral rectus (cut)

superior orbital fissure

Figure 8.2   Course of the oculomotor nerve

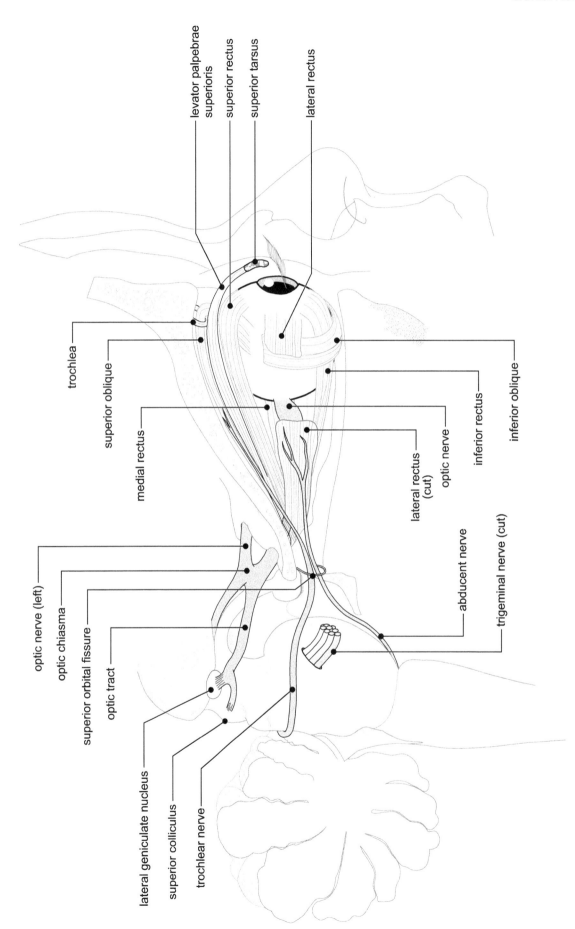

levator palpebrae superioris

superior rectus

superior tarsus

lateral rectus

trochlea

superior oblique

medial rectus

inferior oblique

inferior rectus

optic nerve

lateral rectus (cut)

abducent nerve

trigeminal nerve (cut)

optic nerve (left)

optic chiasma

superior orbital fissure

optic tract

lateral geniculate nucleus

superior colliculus

trochlear nerve

Figure 8.3 Course of the optic, trochlear and abducent nerves

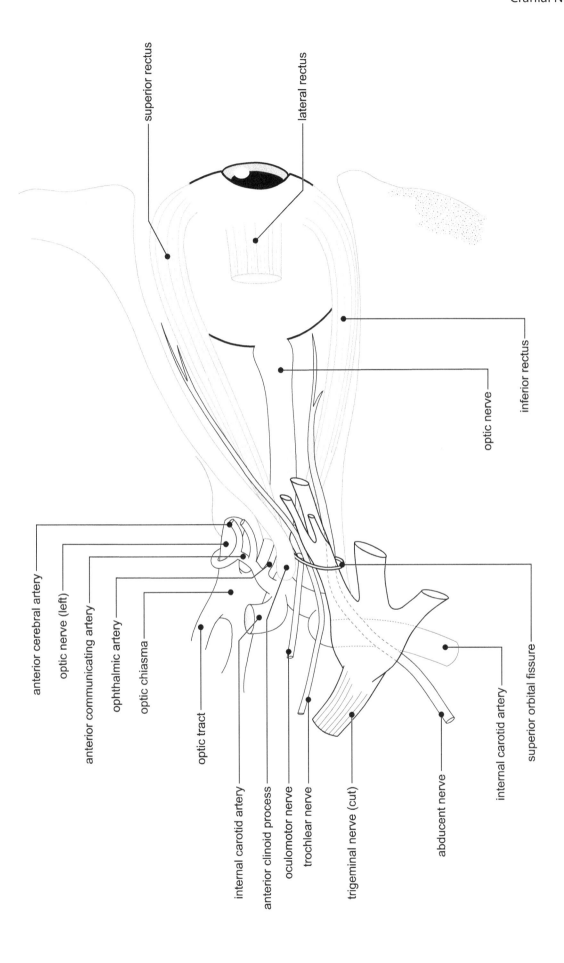

superior rectus

lateral rectus

optic nerve

inferior rectus

anterior cerebral artery

optic nerve (left)

anterior communicating artery

ophthalmic artery

optic chiasma

optic tract

internal carotid artery

anterior clinoid process

oculomotor nerve

trochlear nerve

trigeminal nerve (cut)

abducent nerve

internal carotid artery

superior orbital fissure

Figure 8.4   Nerves and arteries of the right orbit

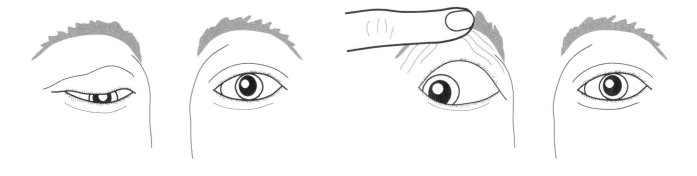

Ptosis (right eye)

Dilation of pupil and lateral strabismus (right eye)

Figure 8.5   Oculomotor nerve palsy

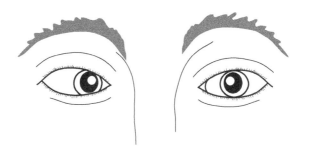

Medial strabismus (right eye)

Figure 8.6   Abducent nerve palsy

4. Ocular Reflexes:

The accommodation and light reflexes involve the oculomotor and optic nerves.

a. **Accommodation reflex** involves convergence, pupil constriction and increase convexity of the lens to focus on a near object. The pathway is indicated as follows:

- from the occipital cortex via corticotectal fibers to:
  - ⇒ superior colliculus
  - ⇒ synapse in *Edinger-Westphal nucleus*
  - ⇒ preganglionic fibers via the oculomotor nerve
  - ⇒ synapse in ciliary ganglion
  - ⇒ postganglionic fibers supply the ***ciliary muscle*** increasing the convexity of the lens for focusing and to the ***sphincter pupillae*** for constriction of the pupil.

b. **Pupillary and Consensual light reflex:**

The pupillary and consensual light reflexes are elicited by shining a light into one eye. The ***pupillary light reflex*** is constriction of the pupil in the eye directly stimulated by the light. The ***consensual light reflex*** is constriction of the pupil in the contralateral eye. The pathway is indicated in Figure 8.7 and is as follows:

From the Retina fibers travel:
- ⇒ via the optic nerve and optic tract
- ⇒ via superior brachium
- ⇒ synapse in *olivary pretectal nucleus*
- ⇒ fibers terminate in the ipsilateral *Edinger-Westphal nucleus*, some fibers pass through the posterior commissure to the contralateral *Edinger-Westphal nucleus*
- ⇒ preganglionic fibers travel via the oculomotor nerves
- ⇒ synapse in the ipsilateral and contralateral ciliary ganglion
- ⇒ postganglionic fibers supply the sphincter pupillae of both eyes to constrict the pupil of the ipsilateral eye, referred to as the ***pupillary light reflex*** and constriction of the contralateral eye, referred to as ***consensual light reflex***

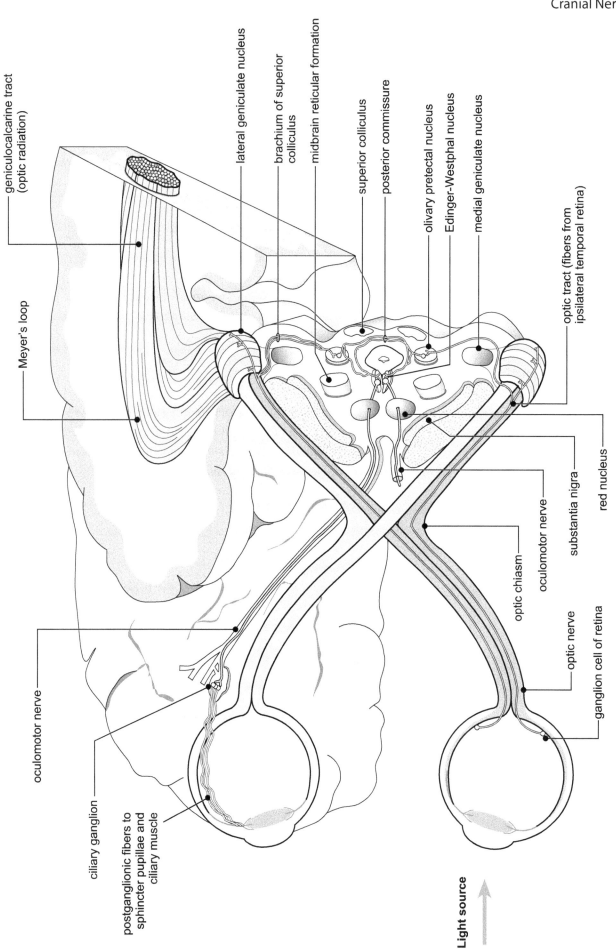

geniculocalcarine tract (optic radiation)

Meyer's loop

lateral geniculate nucleus

brachium of superior colliculus

midbrain reticular formation

superior colliculus

posterior commissure

olivary pretectal nucleus

Edinger-Westphal nucleus

medial geniculate nucleus

optic tract (fibers from ipsilateral temporal retina)

red nucleus

substantia nigra

oculomotor nerve

optic chiasm

optic nerve

ganglion cell of retina

oculomotor nerve

ciliary ganglion

postganglionic fibers to sphincter pupillae and ciliary muscle

Light source

Figure 8.7   Pathway mediating the pupillary light reflex

B. Trigeminal Nerve:

The trigeminal nerve is a mixed nerve containing sensory and motor fibers. It transmits sensory information from the face and supplies muscles of mastication.

1. General features:

- cell bodies of sensory neurons are located in the ***trigeminal ganglion***
- peripheral processes of sensory neurons in the ***trigeminal ganglion*** form three divisions. These are the: ***ophthalmic nerve***, ***maxillary nerve*** and ***mandibular nerve*** (Figure 8.8). The mandibular nerve also has a motor component.
- the central branches of the three divisions join to form a large ***sensory root***, proximal to the trigeminal ganglion. Motor fibers exit through the ***motor root.***

2. Innervation (Figure 8.8):

- the ***ophthalmic nerve*** mediates sensation from the forehead, scalp and nasal mucosa
- the ***maxillary nerve*** mediates sensation from the upper jaw area and upper teeth
- the ***mandibular nerve*** mediates sensation from the lower jaw, lower teeth, cheek and tongue. It also contains motor fibers that supply the muscles of mastication

3. Nuclei:

There are three sensory nuclei and one motor nuclei. The following description is restricted to the general features of the various nuclei. These are indicated in Figure 8.1 and include the following:

a. ***spinal trigeminal nucleus***:
   - is located in the tegmentum of the medulla and pons, extending to level of C3
   - conveys pain, temperature, light touch

b. ***pontine trigeminal nucleus***:
   - is located in the pontine tegmentum
   - conveys fine touch, pressure

c. ***mesencephalic nucleus***:
   - is located in the midbrain and pontine tegmentum
   - consists of unipolar sensory neurons, and is the only example of sensory neurons located in the CNS rather than its usual location in the dorsal root ganglia
   - conveys proprioception

d. ***trigeminal motor nucleus***:
   - is located in the pontine tegmentum
   - supplies muscles of mastication

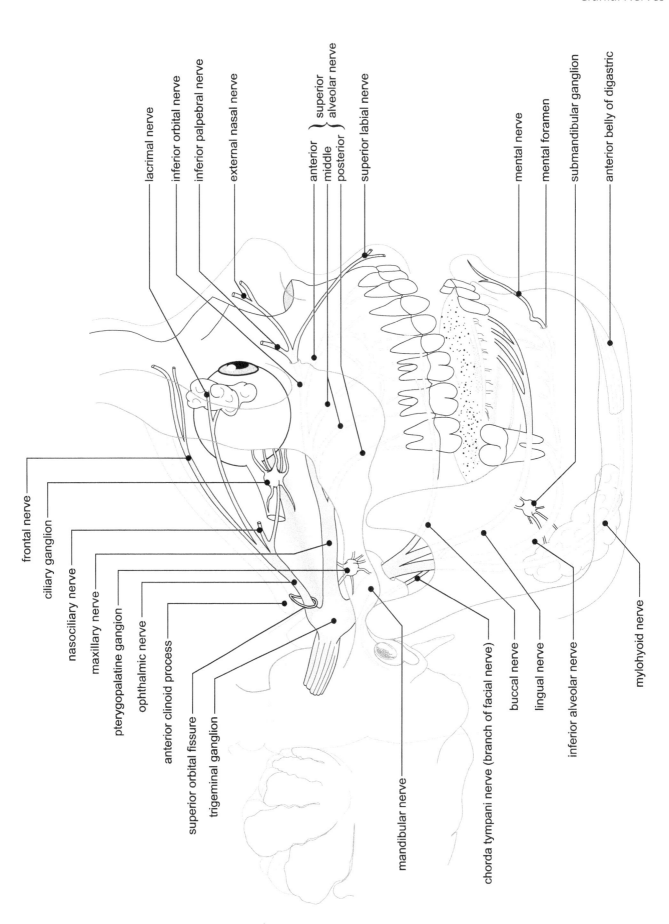
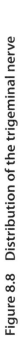

lacrimal nerve

inferior orbital nerve

inferior palpebral nerve

external nasal nerve

anterior } superior
middle   } alveolar nerve
posterior }

superior labial nerve

mental nerve

mental foramen

submandibular ganglion

anterior belly of digastric

frontal nerve

ciliary ganglion

nasociliary nerve

maxillary nerve

pterygopalatine ganglion

ophthalmic nerve

anterior clinoid process

superior orbital fissure

trigeminal ganglion

mandibular nerve

chorda tympani nerve (branch of facial nerve)

buccal nerve

lingual nerve

inferior alveolar nerve

mylohyoid nerve

Figure 8.8   Distribution of the trigeminal nerve

4. *Pathways and Functions:*

I. ***General Somatic Afferent Pathways*** (Figure 8.9):

a. ***Pain, temperature and light touch*** is conveyed from areas of the face:

via the divisions of trigeminal nerve to:

⟹ the trigeminal ganglion (primary sensory neurons)
⟹ via sensory root
⟹ fibers form the ***spinal trigeminal tract***
⟹ synapse in *spinal trigeminal nucleus*
⟹ fibers cross in medulla
⟹ forms the **ventral trigeminothalamic tract**
⟹ ascends through the tegmentum of pons, midbrain
⟹ synapse in the ventral posterior medial nucleus of the thalamus
⟹ relays in the primary sensory area of the cerebral cortex

b. **Fine touch and pressure** is conveyed from areas of the face:

via the divisions of trigeminal nerve to:

⟹ the trigeminal ganglion (primary sensory neurons)
⟹ sensory root
⟹ forms the spinal trigeminal tract
⟹ synapses in ***spinal trigeminal nucleus*** and ***pontine trigeminal nucleus***
⟹ efferent fibers from these nuclei ascend ipsilaterally and contralaterally fibers in the medulla to form the **ventral trigeminothalamic tract** and the **dorsal trigeminothalamic tract**
⟹ ascends in the tegmentum of the pons, midbrain
⟹ synapses in the ventral posterior medial nucleus of the thalamus
⟹ relays to the primary sensory area in the cerebral cortex

c. **Proprioception** is conveyed from (Figure 8.10):

i. proprioceptors adjacent to the teeth of lower jaw/upper jaw
ii. neuromuscular spindles in the muscles of mastication

• via mandibular and maxillary divisions of the trigeminal nerve to:

⟹ trigeminal ganglion
⟹ peripheral branches of the *primary sensory neurons* of the **mesencephalic nucleus** form the ***mesencephalic tract***

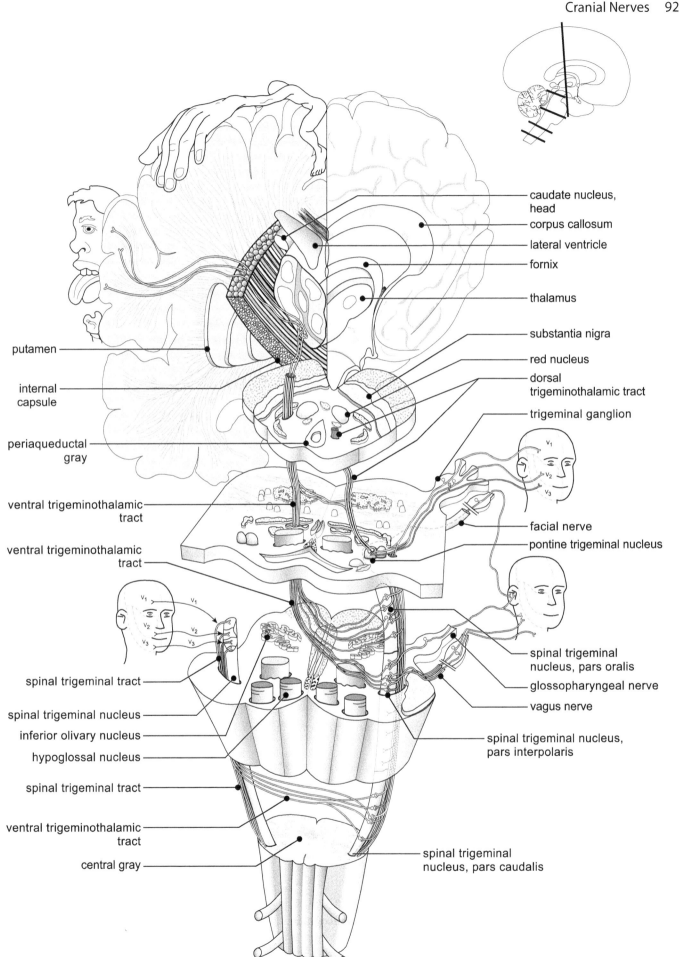

caudate nucleus, head

corpus callosum

lateral ventricle

fornix

thalamus

substantia nigra

red nucleus

dorsal trigeminothalamic tract

trigeminal ganglion

facial nerve

pontine trigeminal nucleus

spinal trigeminal nucleus, pars oralis

glossopharyngeal nerve

vagus nerve

spinal trigeminal nucleus, pars interpolaris

spinal trigeminal nucleus, pars caudalis

putamen

internal capsule

periaqueductal gray

ventral trigeminothalamic tract

ventral trigeminothalamic tract

spinal trigeminal tract

spinal trigeminal nucleus

inferior olivary nucleus

hypoglossal nucleus

spinal trigeminal tract

ventral trigeminothalamic tract

central gray

Figure 8.9   Pathways mediating sensory information from the face

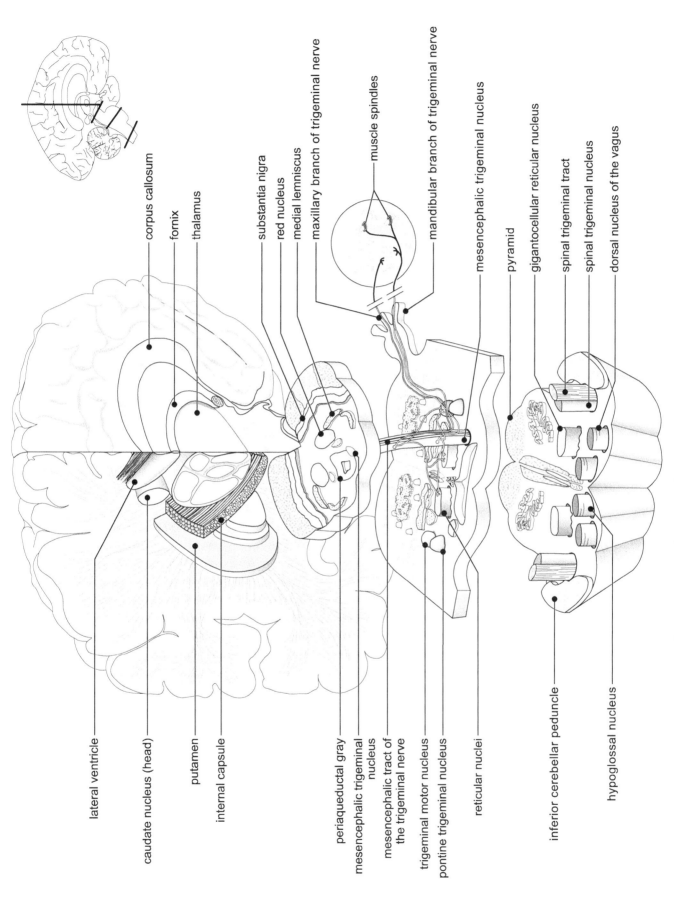

Figure 8.10 Pathway mediating proprioception from the face

lateral ventricle

caudate nucleus (head)

putamen

internal capsule

corpus callosum

fornix

thalamus

substantia nigra

red nucleus

medial lemniscus

maxillary branch of trigeminal nerve

muscle spindles

mandibular branch of trigeminal nerve

mesencephalic trigeminal nucleus

pyramid

gigantocellular reticular nucleus

spinal trigeminal tract

spinal trigeminal nucleus

dorsal nucleus of the vagus

periaqueductal gray

mesencephalic trigeminal nucleus

mesencephalic tract of the trigeminal nerve

trigeminal motor nucleus

pontine trigeminal nucleus

reticular nuclei

inferior cerebellar peduncle

hypoglossal nucleus

⇒ central branches synapse in the trigeminal motor nucleus to supply muscles of mastication

⇒ for reflex control of force of bite

Clinical Notes:

 i. ***Trigeminal neuralgia* (*tic douloureux*)**

  • caused by demyelination of axons in the sensory root, possibly as a result of pressure of a blood vessel on the nerve

  • results in attacks of severe pain over areas supplied by the maxillary and mandibular nerves

 ii. ***Herpes zoster* (*shingles*)**

  • viral infection, affecting neurons in the trigeminal ganglion resulting in painful skin eruptions in the area supplied by branches of the trigeminal nerve

II. *Motor Innervation*:

Trigeminal motor nucleus:

 • axons enter the motor root, travel through the mandibular nerve to supply the masseter, temporalis, pterygoid and several small muscles

Clinical Notes:

Lesion of the trigeminal motor nucleus or motor root of the trigeminal nerve causes weakness of muscles of mastication. There is ipsilateral deviation of the jaw during chewing (Figure 8.11)

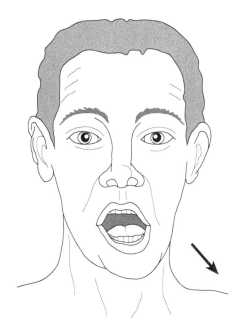

Figure 8.11   Trigeminal nerve lesion

C. Facial Nerve:

The facial nerve is a mixed nerve containing sensory and motor fibers. The facial nerve mediates taste from the anterior two-thirds of the tongue, supplies facial muscles and contains parasympathetic efferents to the lacrimal, submandibular and sublingual glands.

1. General features:

- cell bodies of sensory neurons are located in the ***geniculate ganglion*** (Figure 8.9)
- central branches of sensory neurons form the ***sensory root*** (***nervus intermedius***), proximal to the geniculate ganglion. Motor fibers exit through the ***motor root.***
- the facial nerve passes through the internal acoustic meatus, runs through the middle ear, travels through the facial canal and emerges through the stylomastoid foramen and terminates into five branches to supply the facial muscles

2. Nuclei, Pathways and Functions:

   I. ***General Somatic Afferents*** (8.9):

      i. ***Pain, temperature and light touch*** is conveyed from the auricle and external auditory meatus:

         - via the facial nerve through:

            ⇒ geniculate ganglion
            ⇒ nervus intermedius
            ⇒ join fibers of the spinal trigeminal tract and terminate in the ***spinal trigeminal nucleus***.

      This pathway is similar to that described for the general somatic afferent pathway for the trigeminal nerve. Refer to Figure 8.9 to review this pathway. In this manner, sensory information is transmitted to the cerebral cortex via the trigeminal system.

   II. ***Special Visceral Afferents:***

      a. ***Taste***: is conveyed from the anterior two-thirds of tongue

         i. ***Nucleus*** (Figure 8.1):
           - **gustatory nucleus:** is the upper part of the **solitary nucleus**, located in the medullary tegmentum

ii. **Pathway** (Figure 8.13):
- from anterior two-thirds of the tongue, via peripheral branches of sensory neurons in geniculate ganglion
⇒ geniculate ganglion
⇒ via central branches of sensory neurons in the geniculate ganglion
⇒ fibers form the *tractus solitarius*
⇒ synapse in **gustatory nucleus**
⇒ axons form the central tegmental tract
⇒ ascend through the tegmentum of the brainstem
⇒ synapse in ventral posterior medial nucleus of the thalamus
⇒ relay in inferior part of the somesthetic area of the cortex and the insula

III. *General Somatic Efferents*:

Innervation of muscles:

1. *Nucleus:*

a. *facial motor nucleus:*
- located in ventrolateral pontine tegmentum (Figure 8.1)
- axons from the facial motor nucleus form the motor root to supply muscles of the face
- the dorsal part of the facial motor nucleus receive bilateral corticonuclear fibers, therefore muscles of the upper part of the face are not affected by a lesion of the frontal cortex. The ventral part of the facial motor nucleus receive contralateral corticonuclear fibers. A lesion of the cerebral cortex will affect the contralateral lower facial muscles

Clinical Notes:
A **lower motor neuron lesion** involving the facial motor nucleus or the peripheral branches of the facial nerve results in ipsilateral facial paralysis or *Bell's palsy*. The affected eye cannot close, there is absence of wrinkles and the corner of the mouth droops on the affected side (Figure 8.14). An **upper motor neuron lesion** involving a unilateral lesion of the corticonuclear fibers results in paralysis of the contralateral lower face. The facial muscles of the upper half of the face are unaffected.

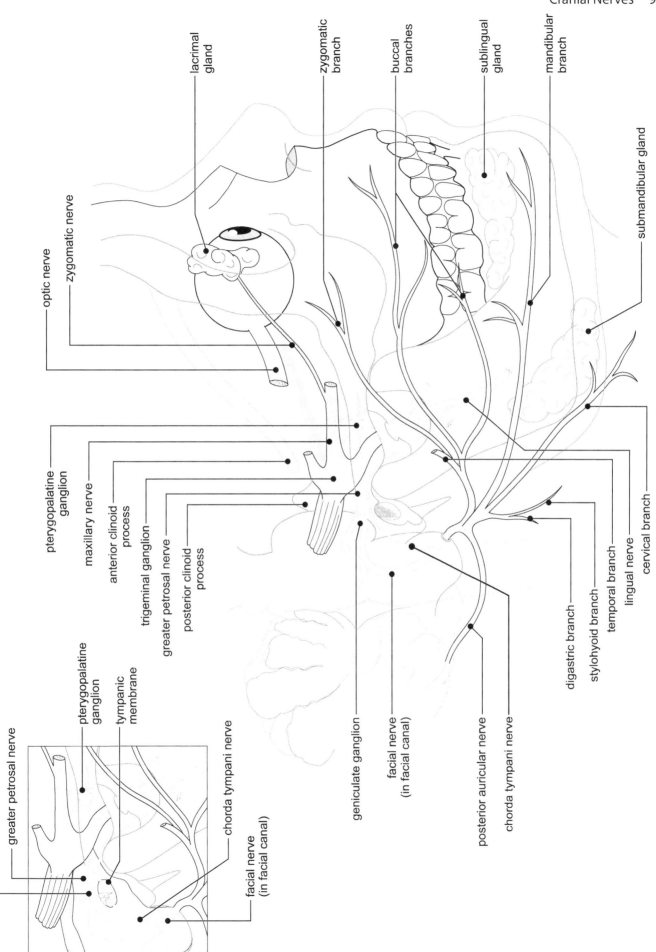

lacrimal gland

zygomatic branch

buccal branches

sublingual gland

mandibular branch

submandibular gland

optic nerve

zygomatic nerve

pterygopalatine ganglion

maxillary nerve

anterior clinoid process

trigeminal ganglion

greater petrosal nerve

posterior clinoid process

geniculate ganglion

facial nerve (in facial canal)

posterior auricular nerve

chorda tympani nerve

digastric branch

stylohyoid branch

temporal branch

lingual nerve

cervical branch

geniculate ganglion

greater petrosal nerve

pterygopalatine ganglion

tympanic membrane

chorda tympani nerve

facial nerve (in facial canal)

Figure 8.12   Distribution of the facial nerve

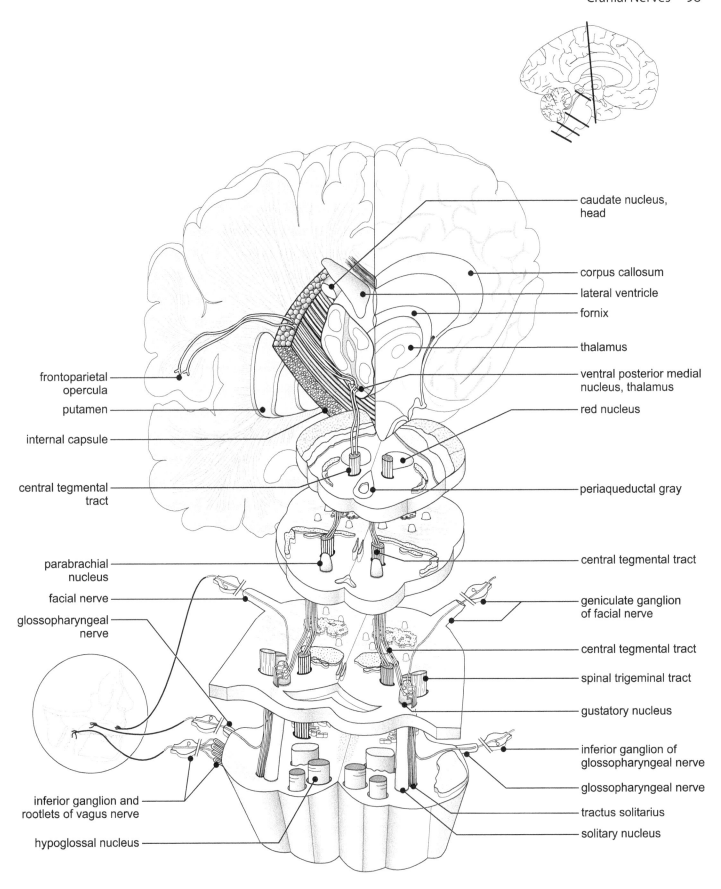

caudate nucleus, head

corpus callosum

lateral ventricle

fornix

thalamus

ventral posterior medial nucleus, thalamus

red nucleus

frontoparietal opercula

putamen

internal capsule

central tegmental tract

periaqueductal gray

central tegmental tract

parabrachial nucleus

facial nerve

glossopharyngeal nerve

geniculate ganglion of facial nerve

central tegmental tract

spinal trigeminal tract

gustatory nucleus

inferior ganglion of glossopharyngeal nerve

glossopharyngeal nerve

inferior ganglion and rootlets of vagus nerve

hypoglossal nucleus

tractus solitarius

solitary nucleus

Figure 8.13   Central pathways mediating taste sensation

IV. *General Visceral Efferents*:

    a. *Parasympathetic components*:

        i. *Nucleus*:

            a. ***superior salivatory nucleus:***
- located in the pontine tegmentum
- axons travel via the facial nerve to supply the ***submandibular*** and ***sublingual glands***

            b. *lacrimal nucleus*:
- is located in the pontine tegmentum
- axons travel via the facial nerve to supply the ***lacrimal gland***

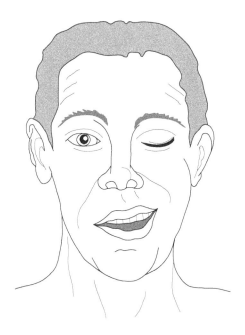

Figure 8.14   Bell's palsy

D. Glossopharyngeal and Vagus nerves

The glossopharyngeal and vagus nerves are similar in both anatomical and functional capabilities and will be described together. The glossopharyngeal and vagus nerves are mixed nerves containing motor, sensory and parasympathetic fibers (Figures 8.15). The vagus nerve has a more extensive distribution, innervating thoracic and abdominal viscera (Figures 8.16 and 8.17).

1. *General Features:*

Each nerve as it exits the skull consists of a ***superior ganglion*** and an ***inferior ganglion***. The superior ganglion contains cell bodies of sensory neurons associated with somatic afferents. The inferior ganglion contains cell bodies of sensory neurons associated with visceral afferents

2. *Nuclei:*

Refer to Figure 8.1 for the locations of the following nuclei:

    a. **gustatory nucleus** – upper part of the solitary nucleus
    b. ***solitary nucleus***:
        • located in tegmentum of medulla
    c. ***nucleus ambiguus***
        • located in the medulla, dorsal to the inferior olivary nucleus

3. *Pathways and Functions*

    I. ***General Somatic Afferents***:

        a. ***Pain, temperature and light touch*** is conveyed from the:

            i. posterior third of the tongue, pharynx and middle ear via the ***glossopharyngeal nerve***
           ii. pharynx, larynx and esophagus via the ***vagus nerve***

           ⇒ information is conveyed via central branches of sensory neurons in the *superior ganglion* of the glossopharyngeal or vagus nerves
           ⇒ fibers join the ***spinal trigeminal tract*** and terminates in the ***spinal trigeminal nucleus***.

This pathway is similar to that described for the general somatic afferent pathway for the trigeminal nerve. Refer to Figure 8.9 to review this pathway. In this manner, sensory information is transmitted to the cerebral cortex via the trigeminal system.

II. *Special Visceral Afferents:*

Taste is conveyed from:
a. posterior 1/3 of tongue via the ***glossopharyngeal nerve***
b. from the epiglottis via the ***vagus nerve***

i. *Nucleus* (Figure 8.1):
- **gustatory nucleus:** is upper part of the **solitary nucleus**, located in the medullary tegmentum

ii. **Pathway** (Figure 8.13):

⇒ information conveyed via central branches of sensory neurons in the inferior ganglion of the glossopharyngeal or vagus nerves joins fibers of the ***solitary tract*** and terminates in the ***gustatory nucleus***. The ascending pathway for taste is illustrated in Figure 8.13 and described in conjunction with the special visceral afferent pathway for the facial nerve.

III. *General Visceral Afferents:*

Reflex control of respiration (by chemoreceptors), blood pressure (by baroreceptors) and digestive functions are mediated as follows:

Input from:
i. baroreceptors in wall of the carotid sinus and chemoreceptors of the carotid body are conveyed via the ***glossopharyngeal nerve***
ii. baroreceptors in the wall of the aortic arch and chemoreceptors of aortic bodies are conveyed via the ***vagus nerve***
iii. thoracic and abdominal viscera (regulatory sensation) via the ***vagus nerve***

Pathway:
⇒ via solitary tract (tractus solitarius)
⇒ synapse in caudal part of nucleus of tractus solitarius
⇒ axons of the solitary nucleus synapse in the dorsal nucleus of the vagus and nucleus ambiguus to decrease heart rate

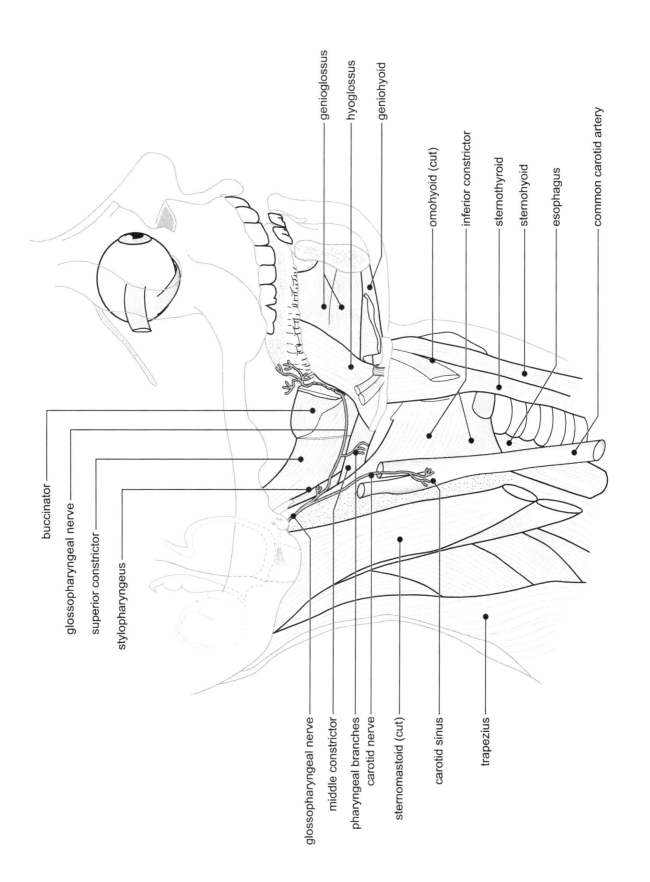

genioglossus

hyoglossus

geniohyoid

omohyoid (cut)

inferior constrictor

sternothyroid

sternohyoid

esophagus

common carotid artery

buccinator

glossopharyngeal nerve

superior constrictor

stylopharyngeus

glossopharyngeal nerve

middle constrictor

pharyngeal branches

carotid nerve

sternomastoid (cut)

carotid sinus

trapezius

Figure 8.15   Distribution of the glossopharyngeal nerve

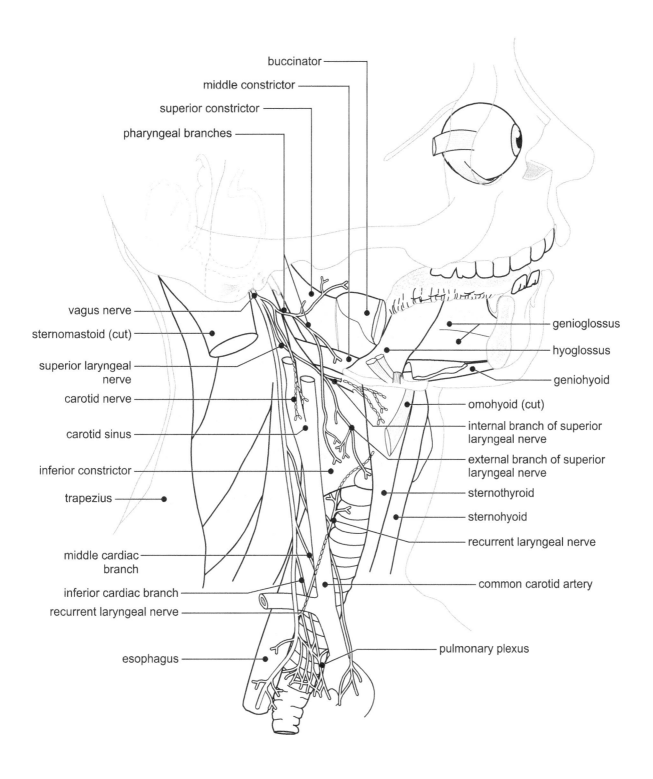

Figure 8.16   Distribution of the vagus nerve

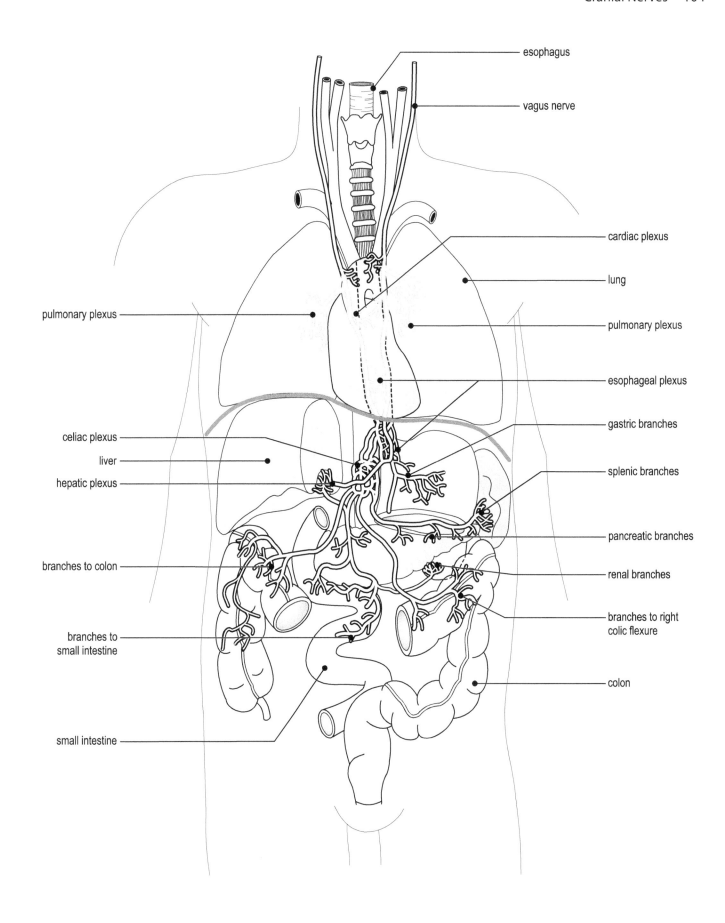

Figure 8.17   Course of the vagus nerve in the thorax and abdomen

⇒ axons of the solitary nucleus synapse in the respiratory centers of the reticular formation and via the reticulospinal tracts synapse in motor neurons of the cervical cord, bringing about contraction of the diaphragm to increase respiration.

IV. *General Somatic Efferents*:

Innervation of muscles:

Nuclei:

i. ***nucleus ambiguus***, *rostral part*, axons join the ***glossopharyngeal nerve*** to supply the stylopharyngeus muscle
ii. ***nucleus ambiguus***, *from a large area of the nucleus*, axons join the ***vagus nerve*** to supply the muscles of the pharynx and esophagus.

V. *General Visceral Efferents*:

a. *Parasympathetic components*:

Nuclei (Figure 8.1)
i. ***inferior salivatory nucleus*** - in medulla
   • axons join the ***glossopharyngeal nerve*** to supply the parotid gland
ii. ***dorsal nucleus of the vagus*** - in vagal trigone in the floor of the fourth ventricle
   • axons join the ***vagus nerve*** and terminate in thoracic and abdominal viscera. The main functions are bronchoconstriction, peristalsis, increase in secretions of the stomach, pancreas and intestine
iii. ***nucleus ambiguus*** - in medulla
   • axons join the ***vagus nerve*** to terminate in the heart to control heart rate

E. Accessory Nerve:

1. General Features:

The accessory nerve is a motor nerve. It is often described as consisting of two components, a ***cranial portion*** and a ***spinal portion***.

2. Nuclei:

a. ***nucleus ambiguus***, *caudal part:* axons form the ***cranial root of the accessory nerve***, which joins the vagus nerve to supply the soft palate and intrinsic muscles of the larynx.
b. ***accessory nucleus***: located in ventral gray horn of C1-C5 segments of the spinal cord (Figures 7.4, 8.1).

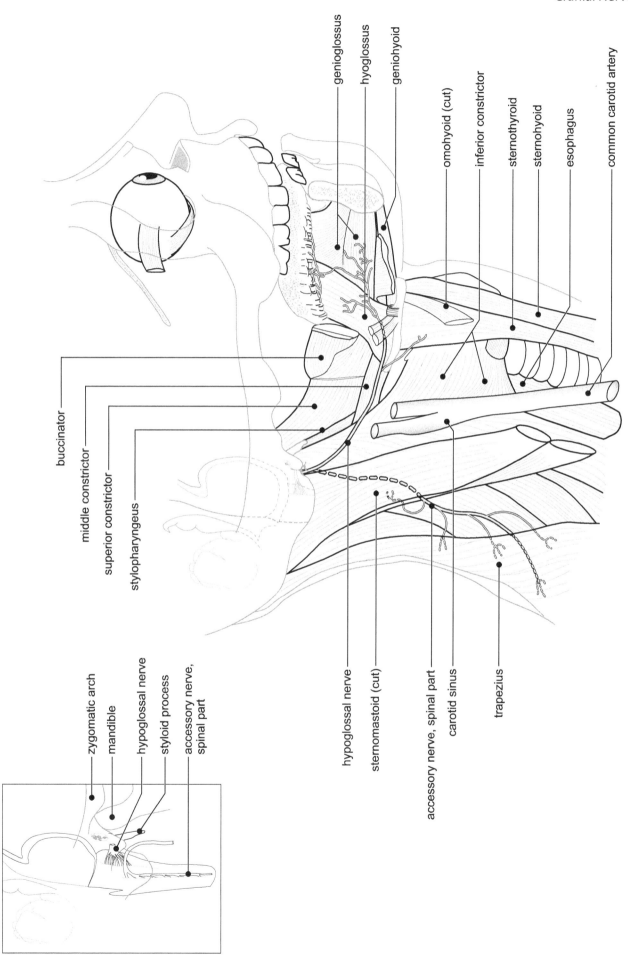

Figure 8.18   Course of the accessory and hypoglossal nerves

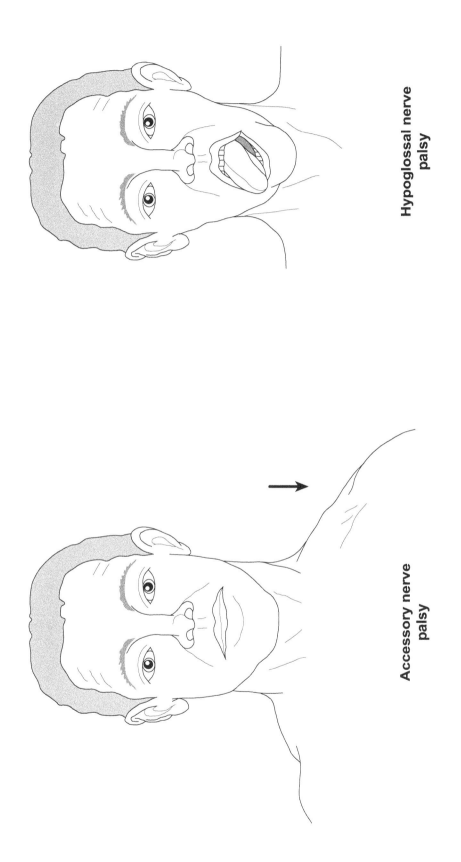

Hypoglossal nerve palsy

Accessory nerve palsy

Figure 8.19   Lesion of the spinal accessory nerve and hypoglossal nerve

3. Pathway:

- axons from the ***accessory nucleus*** form the ***spinal root*** of the accessory nerve (Figure 7.4). The spinal root of the accessory nerve ascends through the foramen magnum, joins the cranial root of the accessory nerve and continues as the accessory nerve as far as the jugular foramen.
- the accessory nerve exits through the jugular foramen and the cranial root separates from the spinal root and joins the vagus nerve.
- the spinal root supplies the trapezius and sternocleidomastoid muscles (Figure 8.18).

Clinical Notes:
Injury to the spinal root of the accessory nerve causes difficulty in raising the shoulder or turning the head to the opposite side (Figure 8.19).

F. Hypoglossal Nerve:

1. General Features:

The hypoglossal nerve is a motor nerve. It supplies the extrinsic and intrinsic muscles of the tongue

1. Nucleus:

a. *hypoglossal nucleus*:
- is located in the hypoglossal trigone, in the floor of the fourth ventricle (Figures 7.4 and 8.1)
- axons from neurons of the hypoglossal nucleus form the hypoglossal nerve.
- the hypoglossal nerve supplies intrinsic and some extrinsic muscles of the tongue (Figure 8.18)
- the hypoglossal nucleus receive ***corticonuclear fibers*** that originate predominantly from the contralateral motor cortex.

Clinical Notes:
i. an unilateral injury to the hypoglossal nucleus or hypoglossal nerve results in a ***lower motor neuron*** lesion. The ipsilateral tongue is paralyzed and flaccid and eventually becomes atrophied. On protrusion, the tongue deviates to the side of the lesion (Figure 8.19)

ii. an unilateral lesion of the corticonuclear fibers results in an ***upper motor neuron*** lesion. The contralateral half of the tongue becomes weak

CHAPTER
9

RETICULAR FORMATION

Overview

The reticular formation consists of a complex network of nuclei, fiber bundles and their connections. The reticular formation forms the core of the brainstem providing a continuum between the diencephalon and the spinal cord. The diffuse aggregation of neurons of the reticular formation are separated from cranial nerve nuclei and tracts in the brainstem. The reticular formation participates in four general types of functions, namely, modulation of sensory input to the cortex, control of consciousness, autonomic regulation and regulation of motor activity.

Only major reticular nuclei and pathways contributing to the four general types of functions will be described in this unit.

I. General Features:

- the reticular formation consists of groups of neurons situated among many fiber bundles in the brainstem tegmentum
- neurons have long branching dendrites, receiving synaptic input from multiple sensory modalities
- neurons have long axons that bifurcate into ascending and descending branches that project to distant areas of the brain

A. Anatomical Organization:

Reticular nuclei are arranged in longitudinal columns of cells, extending from medial to lateral as follows:

Refer to Figure 9.1 for the various groups of nuclei

1. Precerebellar Nuclei:

- are functionally separate from the rest of the reticular nuclei
- projects to the cerebellum and functions in coordination of movement

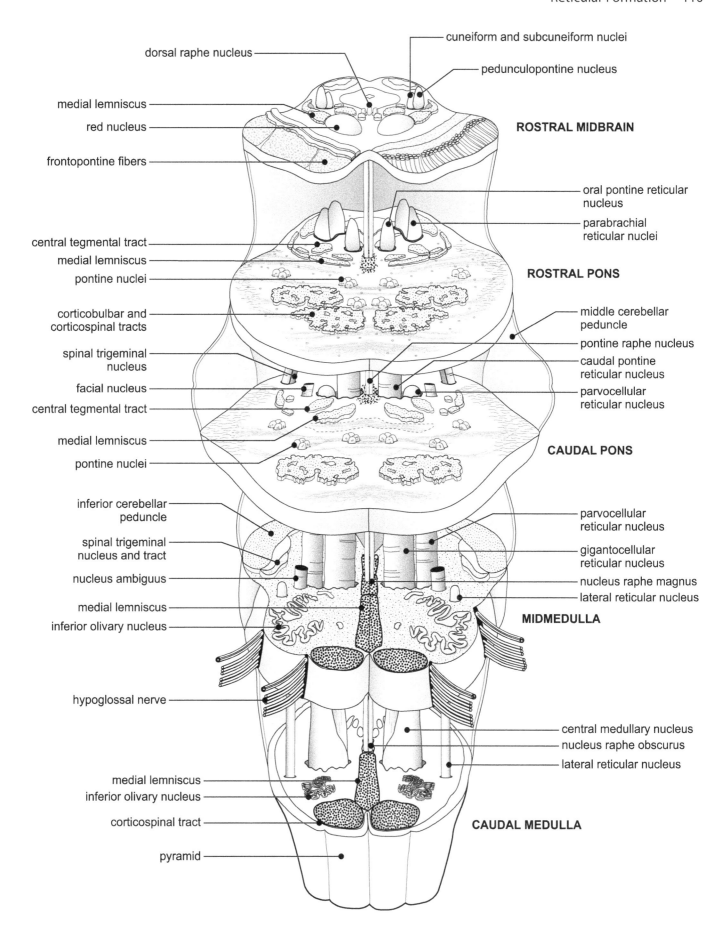

dorsal raphe nucleus

cuneiform and subcuneiform nuclei

pedunculopontine nucleus

medial lemniscus

red nucleus

frontopontine fibers

ROSTRAL MIDBRAIN

oral pontine reticular nucleus

parabrachial reticular nuclei

central tegmental tract

medial lemniscus

pontine nuclei

ROSTRAL PONS

corticobulbar and corticospinal tracts

middle cerebellar peduncle

pontine raphe nucleus

spinal trigeminal nucleus

caudal pontine reticular nucleus

facial nucleus

parvocellular reticular nucleus

central tegmental tract

medial lemniscus

pontine nuclei

CAUDAL PONS

inferior cerebellar peduncle

parvocellular reticular nucleus

spinal trigeminal nucleus and tract

gigantocellular reticular nucleus

nucleus ambiguus

nucleus raphe magnus

lateral reticular nucleus

medial lemniscus

inferior olivary nucleus

MIDMEDULLA

hypoglossal nerve

central medullary nucleus

nucleus raphe obscurus

lateral reticular nucleus

medial lemniscus

inferior olivary nucleus

corticospinal tract

CAUDAL MEDULLA

pyramid

Figure 9.1   Nuclei of the reticular formation

2. Raphe nuclei:

- are narrow plate of neurons located adjacent to the midline
- includes five nuclear groups that extend the entire length of the brainstem
- releases serotonin as the neurotransmitter
- projects to the cerebellum and all parts of the cerebrum
- rostrally projecting neurons are active in sleep
- caudally projecting neurons play a role in modulation of pain

3. Central Reticular nuclei:

- are located lateral to the *Raphe nuclei*
- includes four nuclear groups that extend the length of the pons and the medulla oblongata, and two laterally located nuclear groups in the midbrain
- receives input from various sensory systems, hypothalamus and premotor area of the cerebral cortex

4. Lateral Reticular nuclei:

- are located lateral to the central reticular nuclei
- extends through the medulla oblongata and the pons
- projects to motor nuclei of cranial nerves involved in feeding

5. Other Reticular Nuclei:

- cholinergic and catecholamine nuclear group
- nuclei of the parabrachial area

B. Functional Organization of the Reticular Formation:

Reticular nuclei are involved in four types of function. These are:

1. Regulates activity of the cortex (ascending reticular activating system)
2. Regulates motor control (reticulospinal system)
3. Regulates autonomic functions (respiration, cardiovascular control)
4. Involved in modulation of pain (raphespinal tract)

1. Control of consciousness:

Ascending Reticular Activating System (Figures 9.2 and 9.3)

The ***central group*** of reticular nuclei receive input from various sources. These are:

Afferents:

- hypothalamus; visual information via the superior colliculus; collateral branches from trigeminothalamic, spinothalamic and spinoreticular sensory pathways

Efferents:

- ascending projections from the reticular formation, via the **central tegmental tract**, terminate in the **intralaminar nuclei of the thalamus**, which in turn project to widespread areas of the **cortex**.

function: activity in this pathway is essential for the maintenance of a normal state of *consciousness*.

Clinical Notes:

Bilateral damage to this pathway results in prolonged *coma*.

2. Motor Control

Motor activity is regulated by corticoreticular fibers, pontine reticulospinal tract and medullary reticulospinal tract (Figure 9.5). Connections are indicated in Figure 9.4.

Afferents:

- *corticoreticular fibers* from premotor cortex and supplementary motor cortex descend through the brainstem in conjunction with corticonuclear and corticospinal tracts. Corticoreticular fibers terminate in the central group of reticular nuclei of the pons and medulla

Efferents:

a. the pontine reticular nuclei give rise to the ***pontine (medial) reticulospinal tract***, which descend through the medulla to the ipsilateral ventral funiculus of the spinal cord. Fibers terminate in laminae V11 and V111, to synapse with interneurons thereby influencing motor neurons at all levels of the spinal cord. This pathway stimulates extensors and inhibits flexors of the axial and proximal limb musculature

b. the medullary reticular nuclei give rise to the ***medullary (lateral) reticulospinal tract***, which descend through the medulla to the ipsilateral and contralateral ventrolateral funiculus. Fibers synapse with interneurons and influence motor neurons at all levels of the spinal cord. This pathway stimulates flexors and inhibits extensors of the axial and proximal limb musculature

Collectively, the reticulospinal tracts modulate muscle tone and regulate postural reflexes.

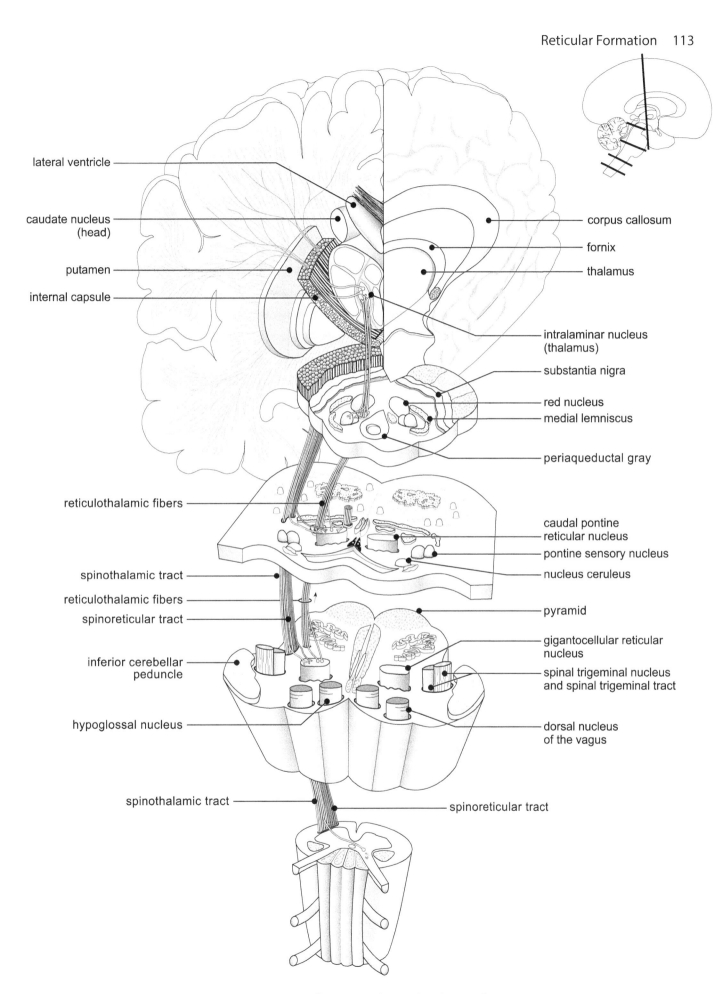

lateral ventricle

caudate nucleus
(head)

putamen

internal capsule

corpus callosum

fornix

thalamus

intralaminar nucleus
(thalamus)

substantia nigra

red nucleus

medial lemniscus

periaqueductal gray

reticulothalamic fibers

caudal pontine
reticular nucleus

pontine sensory nucleus

nucleus ceruleus

spinothalamic tract

reticulothalamic fibers

spinoreticular tract

pyramid

gigantocellular reticular
nucleus

inferior cerebellar
peduncle

spinal trigeminal nucleus
and spinal trigeminal tract

hypoglossal nucleus

dorsal nucleus
of the vagus

spinothalamic tract

spinoreticular tract

Figure 9.2   Ascending reticular activating pathway

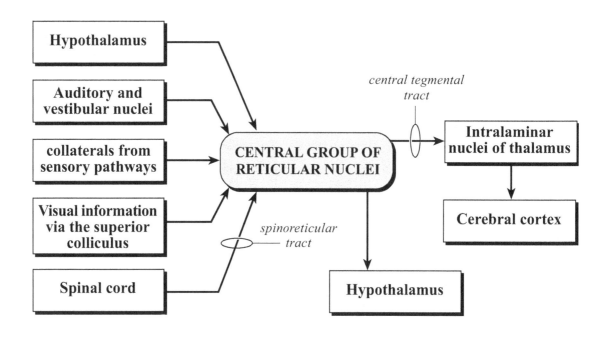

Figure 9.3   Connections of the ascending reticular activating system

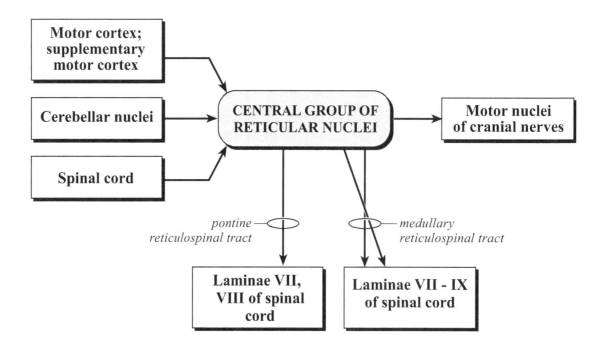

Figure 9.4   Corticoreticular and reticulospinal pathways in motor control

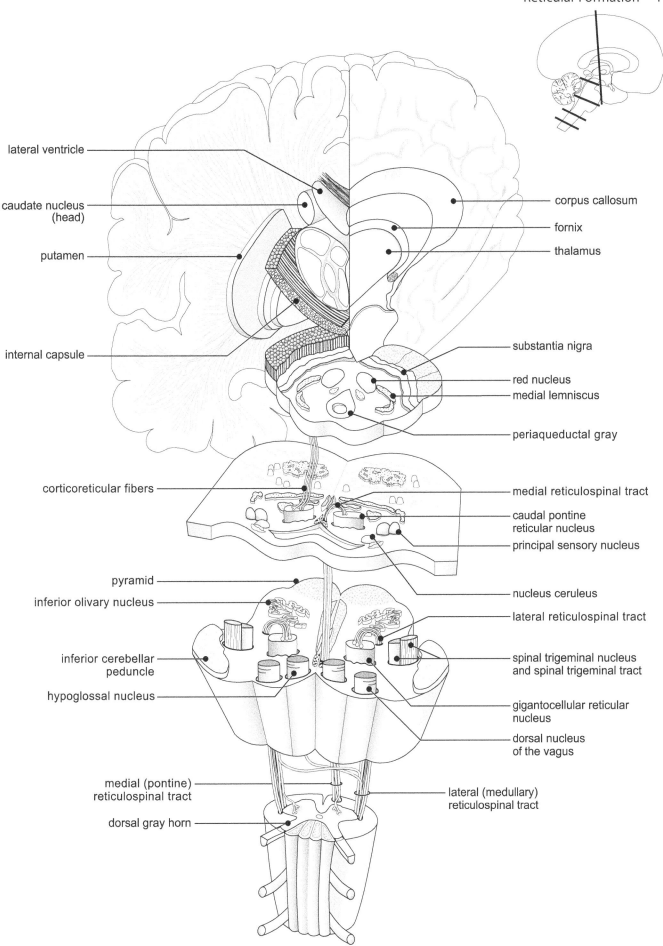

Figure 9.5   Reticulospinal pathways

3. Modulation of Autonomic Functions:

The reticular formation consists of excitatory and inhibitory centers in the medulla and pons that regulate the cardiovascular and respiratory systems.

Cardiovascular Centers consist of the following:
  a. ***excitatory center***: in lateral part of the reticular formation. Stimulation results in increase heart rate and blood pressure.

  b. ***inhibitory center***:
     • is located in the medial part of the reticular formation.
     • stimulation results in decrease heart rate and blood pressure

Respiratory Centers:

  a. ***expiratory center***
     • is located in the lateral part of the reticular formation
     • decreased oxygen concentration in circulating blood results in increase in the rate and depth of breathing, for example, in vigorous exercise.

  b. ***inspiratory center***
     • is located in the medial part of the reticular formation
     • increased levels of carbon dioxide in circulating blood stimulates contraction of diaphragm and intercostal muscles via reticulospinal connections

4. Modulation of Pain:

Descending pathways from the reticular formation modulate perception of pain (Figure 9.6). The physiological control of descending inhibitory pain pathway is as follows:

> During a stressful experience, many areas of the brain, namely the prefrontal cortex, hypothalamus and amygdala project to neurons of the ***periaqueductal gray*** of the midbrain. Neurons of the periaqueductal gray release *enkephalins* and their axons form excitatory synapses with neurons of the ***nucleus raphe magnus*** of the medulla. Raphe nuclei release *serotonin*. Efferents from the nucleus raphe magnus, the ***raphespinal tract*** (Figure 9.6) descend through the brainstem, crosses the dorsal part of the lateral funiculus of the spinal cord and synapses in the substantia gelatinosa of the dorsal gray horn. In response, inhibitory interneurons of the substantia gelatinosa are excited and release *enkephalins*. Enkephalins bind with opiate receptors present at the terminals of sensory neurons of the dorsal root ganglion and tract cells. This results in decrease amounts of *glutamate* or *substance P* being released, thereby inhibiting the transmission of pain via the ascending spinothalamic tract (Figure 9.7).

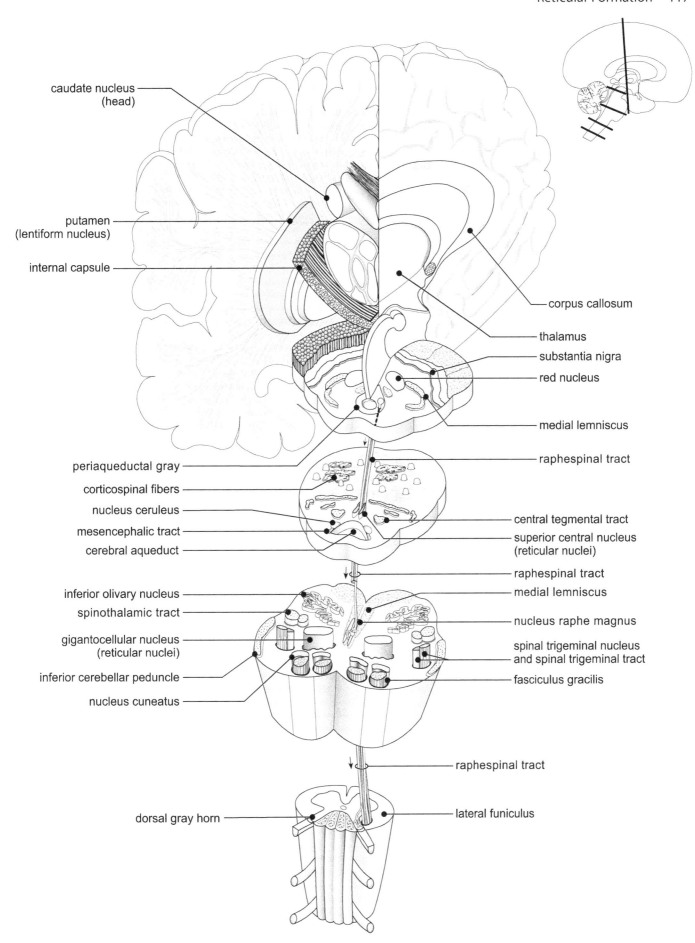

Figure 9.6   Raphespinal pathway

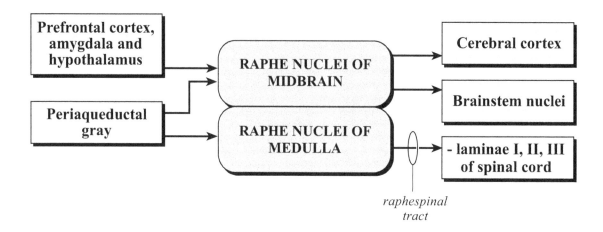

Figure 9.7   Connections of the raphe nuclei involved in the modulation of pain

Gate control theory of Pain:

The gate control theory of pain indicates that impulses conveying pain can be modulated by sensory impulses conveyed from nonpainful sources. For example, massaging a painful area reduces the sensation of pain. Figure 9-8 explains this pathway. Pain conveyed via Aδ and C fibers terminate in the substantia gelatinosa of the dorsal gray horn, inhibit the inhibitory interneuron thereby resulting in activation of tract cells that transmit pain via the spinothalamic tract. By massaging the painful area, Aβ fibers conveying touch stimulate the inhibitory neuron in the substantia gelatinosa of the dorsal gray, which in turn inhibits the activity of tract cells that convey pain through the spinothalamic tract, to keep the "gate closed".

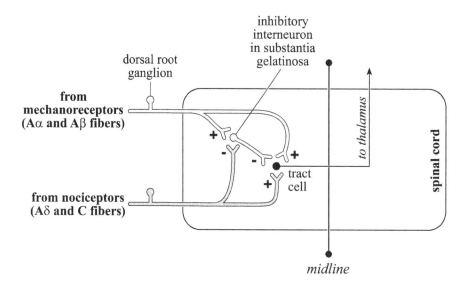

Figure 9.8   Schematic diagram of the gate control theory of pain

CHAPTER
10
_____

CEREBELLUM

Overview

The cerebellum plays an important role in coordination of movement. In general, the cerebellum exerts its influence on the nuclei of the brainstem and thalamus, which in turn regulate the activity of the motor cortex. In this way, the cerebellum is able to compare the intended movement with the movement in progress and allow for a smooth and accurate execution of the desired movement. The cerebellum is also important in maintaining muscle tone, posture and balance.

I. Gross Anatomy:

A. Location:

- located in the floor of the posterior cranial fossa
- separated from the cerebrum by the tentorium cerebelli
- dorsal to the pons and medulla oblongata and forms the roof of the fourth ventricle

B. Features:

- consists of two *cerebellar hemispheres* and a mid portion, the *vermis*. The vermis separates the cerebellar hemispheres and is present on both the superior and inferior surfaces of the hemispheres (Figures 10.1 and 10.2)
- the cerebellum is connected to the midbrain by the *superior cerebellar peduncle*, with the pons by the *middle cerebellar peduncle* and with the medulla oblongata by the *inferior cerebellar peduncle*

C. Fissures and Lobes of the cerebellar hemispheres:

- *dorsolateral fissure*: on the inferior surface, at caudal border of flocculonodular lobe
- *primary fissure*: separates anterior and posterior lobes of the cerebellar hemispheres
- *posterior superior fissure*: on the inferior surface, separates the posterior lobe of cerebellar hemispheres
- *anterior lobe:* on the superior surface of the cerebellar hemispheres, rostral to the primary fissure

- *posterior lobe*: remainder of the cerebellar hemispheres on the superior and inferior surfaces
- *paravermal cortex:* narrow area on the medial side of each cerebellar hemisphere, located lateral to the vermis
- *flocculonodular lobe*: small component at rostral edge of inferior surface of cerebellum and separates the posterior lobe. It consists of the *nodule*, located at the rostral end of the inferior vermis and the *flocculi* on either side of the nodule

II. Internal Structure:

A. Cortex:

- superficial to the white matter, highly convoluted and contained in narrow parallel folds or *folia*, separated by sulci

B. Medullary center:

- forms the internal core of white matter
- consists of afferent and efferent tracts and central cerebellar nuclei

C. Central Cerebellar Nuclei: 4 pairs

1. *Fastigial nucleus*: located in the midline, in contact with the roof of the fourth ventricle

   - efferents travel via inferior cerebellar peduncle $\Rightarrow$ vestibular nuclei

2. *Interposed nucleus*: located lateral to the fastigial nucleus and medial to the dentate nucleus

   - includes the *emboliform nucleus*, located medial to the dentate nucleus, and the *globose nucleus*, located medial to the emboliform nucleus (Figure 15.2)

   - efferents travel via the superior cerebellar peduncle $\Rightarrow$ contralateral red nucleus and ventral lateral (posterior division) nucleus of the thalamus

3. *Dentate nucleus*: largest and most lateral of the central cerebellar nuclei (Figure 15.2)

   - efferents project to the contralateral ventral lateral (posterior division) nucleus of thalamus.

III. Cerebellar Peduncles:

1. *Superior cerebellar peduncle* - predominantly output pathway

   Afferents: ventral spinocerebellar tract; rubrocerebellar tract

   Efferents: cerebellothalamic fibers (to ventral lateral nucleus of the thalamus) and cerebellorubral fibers (to red nucleus)

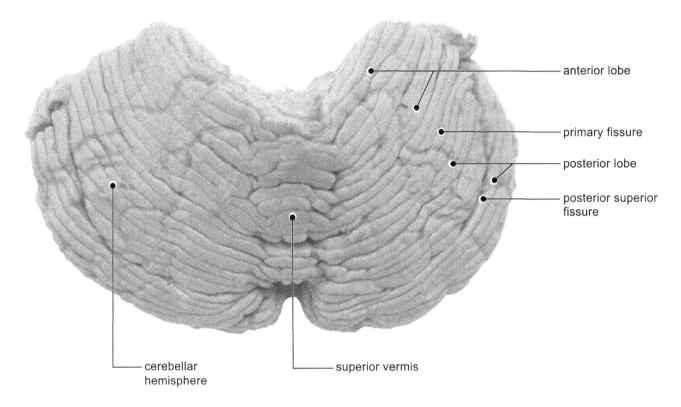

anterior lobe

primary fissure

posterior lobe

posterior superior
fissure

cerebellar
hemisphere

superior vermis

Figure 10.1   Superior surface of the cerebellum

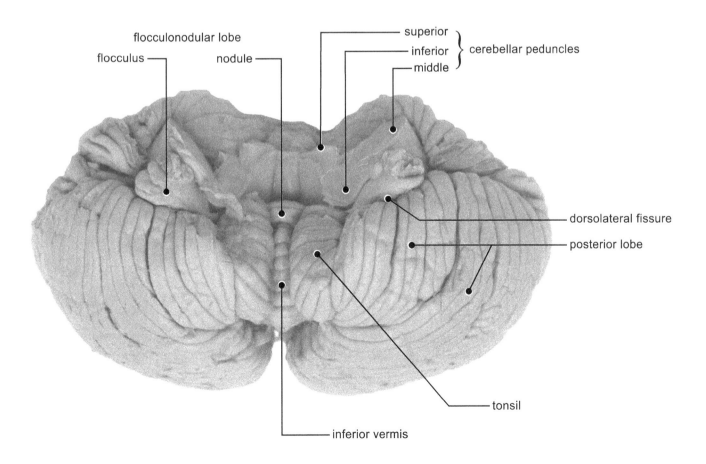

flocculonodular lobe

flocculus

nodule

superior

inferior

middle

cerebellar peduncles

dorsolateral fissure

posterior lobe

tonsil

inferior vermis

Figure 10.2   Inferior surface of the cerebellum

2. *Middle cerebellar peduncle* - input pathway

    Afferents: pontocerebellar fibers

3. *Inferior cerebellar peduncle* - input and output pathways

    Afferents: dorsal spinocerebellar tract, cuneocerebellar tract, olivocerebellar fibers, reticulocerebellar fibers and vestibulocerebellar fibers

    Efferents: cerebellovestibular fibers (to vestibular nuclei) and cerebelloreticular fibers (to reticular nuclei)

IV. Structural Organization:

Consists of 3 cortical layers (Figure 10.3). These are:

1. *Molecular layer*:

    - outer layer of the cortex
    - consists of **stellate cells, basket cells**; purkinje cell dendritic arborizations; **parallel fibers** and **climbing fibers**
    - parallel fibers are axons of granule cells. Parallel fibers run along the surface of the folium and contact many purkinje cells and dendrites of stellate, basket and golgi neurons
    - climbing fibers climb through the dendritic tree of purkinje cells and each fiber contacts one purkinje cell

2. *Purkinje cell layer*:

    - middle cell layer
    - consists of a single layer of **purkinje cells**, the principal neuron of the cerebellum
    - dendritic tree of purkinje cells extend into the molecular layer. The axon of the purkinje cell project to the central nuclei of cerebellum and vestibular nuclei. Purkinje cells are the only efferent neurons of the cerebellar cortex

3. *Granule cell layer*:

    - innermost cell layer
    - consists of **granule cells, golgi cells**; **mossy fibers** and **cerebellar glomerulus**
    - granule cell axons extend to the molecular layer, bifurcate and run parallel to the folia, forming **parallel fibers**. Granule cells are the only excitatory neuron in the cerebellar cortex
    - Each mossy fiber branches and terminates into **rosettes.** A mossy fiber rosette, granule cell dendrites and golgi cell axon form the **glomerulus**

V. Internal Circuitry:

A. Afferent Fibers:

Afferent information enter the cerebellum through two types of fibers, climbing fibers and mossy fibers:

1. ***Climbing fibers*** are afferent excitatory fibers from the contralateral inferior olivary nucleus. Each climbing fiber extends through the granule cell and purkinje cell layers and synapses with dendrites of a purkinje cell (Figure 10.3). The excitatory neurotransmitter is aspartate.

2. ***Mossy fibers*** are excitatory afferent fibers from pontine nuclei and spinocerebellar pathways. Each mossy fiber extends into the granule cell layer, terminate into rosettes and synapse with dendrites of many granule cells. The excitatory neurotransmitter is glutamate.

B. Intracortical circuits:

- Mossy fibers excite granule cells, which in turn excite purkinje cells via parallel fibers. Parallel fibers synapse on dendritic spines of purkinje cells and many parallel fibers are necessary to activate a purkinje cell.   Granule cells, via parallel fibers, also excite stellate, basket and golgi cells.
- A single climbing fiber makes multiple excitatory synapses on the dendritic tree of a single purkinje cell, resulting in prolonged depolarization of the purkinje cell. Activated purkinje cells inhibit groups of neurons of the central cerebellar and vestibular nuclei. The inhibitory neurotransmitter is *GABA.*
- At the same time, purkinje cells that do not lie in the plane of the activated parallel fiber are inhibited by stellate and basket cells. The golgi cell, activated by the parallel fiber, inhibits the granule cell. This results in modulation of the inhibitory action of purkinje cells and a consequent increase in excitation of the central cerebellar nuclei.

C. Summary of Circuitry:

$\oplus$ = excitatory synapses
$\ominus$ = inhibitory synapses

A. INPUT:
- climbing fibers $\Rightarrow$ $\oplus$ purkinje cell dendrites
- mossy fibers $\Rightarrow$ $\oplus$ granule cell

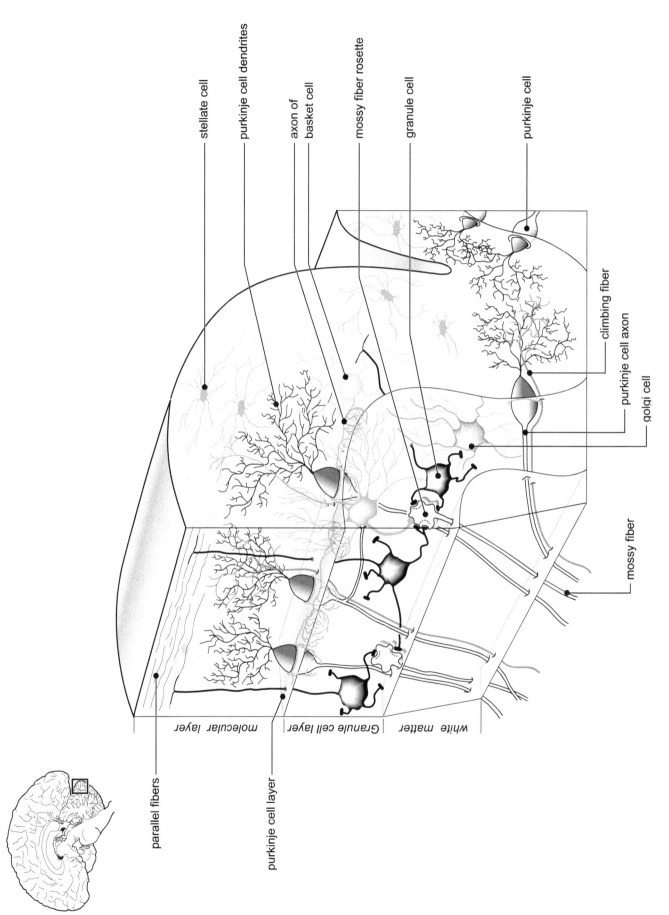

stellate cell

purkinje cell dendrites

axon of
basket cell

mossy fiber rosette

granule cell

purkinje cell

climbing fiber

purkinje cell axon

golgi cell

mossy fiber

molecular layer

Granule cell layer

white matter

parallel fibers

purkinje cell layer

Figure 10.3   Circuitry of the cerebellum

B. INTERNAL:

- basket cell   ⇒ Θ purkinje cell soma
- stellate cell   ⇒ Θ purkinje cell dendrites
- golgi cell   ⇒ Θ granule cell
- purkinje cell   ⇒ Θ golgi cell
- parallel fibers   ⇒ ⊕ purkinje cell dendrites
  (granule cell)   ⇒ ⊕ basket cell and stellate cell dendrites
                      ⇒ ⊕ golgi cell dendrites

C. OUTPUT

- purkinje cell   ⇒ Θ deep cerebellar nuclei
                     ⇒ Θ vestibular nuclei

VI. Divisions of the Cerebellum:

A. With reference to connections and functions, the cerebellum can be combined into three divisions. These are:

1. **Archicerebellum**, also termed the **Vestibulocerebellum**

    Anatomical components: flocculonodular lobe
    Nuclear projection: fastigial nucleus
    Functional significance: regulates muscle tone and equilibrium

2. **Paleocerebellum**, also termed the **Spinocerebellum**

    Anatomical components: superior vermis in the anterior lobe and part of
                            inferior vermis in the posterior lobe; paravermal cortex
    Nuclear projection: interposed nucleus (globose and emboliform nuclei)
    Functional significance: regulates muscle tone and synergy

3. **Neocerebellum**, also termed the **Pontocerebellum**

    Anatomical components: cerebellar hemispheres and superior vermis in
                            posterior lobe
    Nuclear projection: dentate nucleus
    Functional significance: precision, sequencing

VII. Functional Anatomy:

1. *Connections of the Vestibulocerebellum:*

The vestibulocerebellum receives primary input from the vestibular nucleus and sends reciprocal connections to the vestibular nucleus via the inferior cerebellar peduncle. Each fastigial nucleus receives input from the vestibulocerebellum, which in turn projects to the vestibular nuclei and reticular nuclei. Vestibular nuclei connect with extraocular motor nuclei of the cranial nerves. The vestibulospinal and reticulospinal pathways innervate axial and proximal limb muscles. Thus, the vestibulocerebellum controls posture and balance in response to head and eye movements (Figure 10. 4 and Figure 10.5).

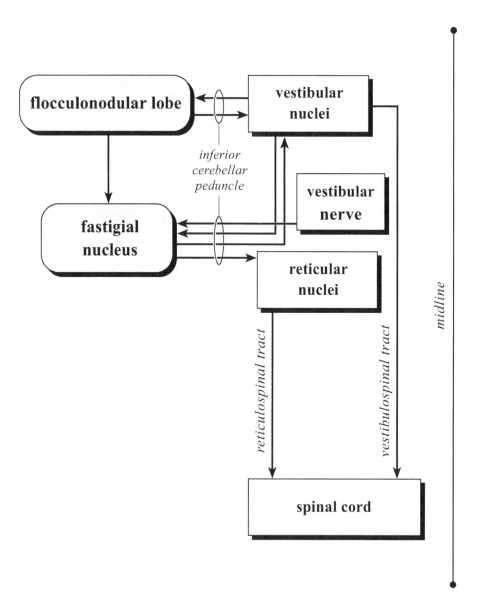

Figure 10.4   Connections of the vestibulocerebellum

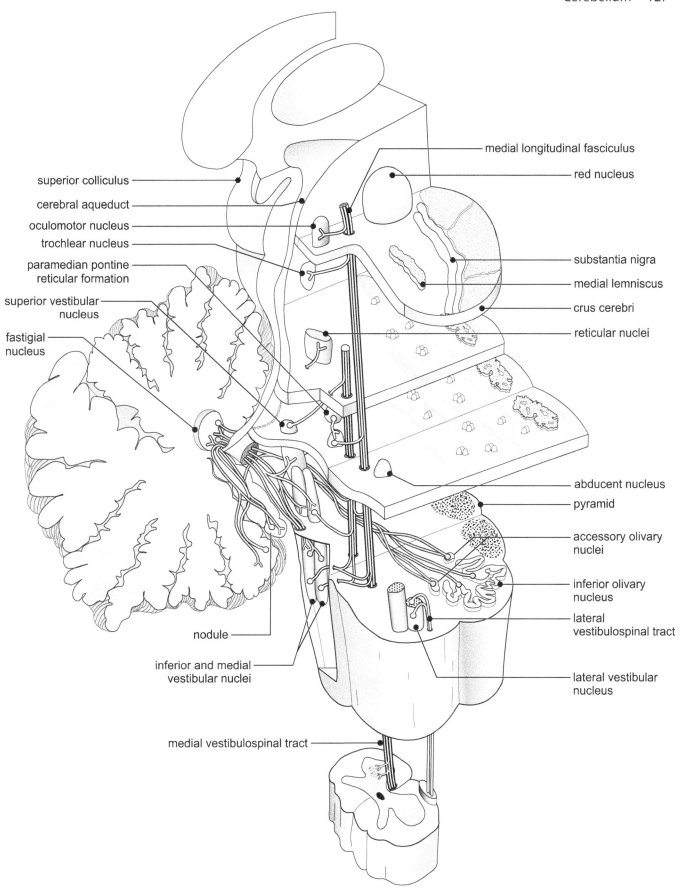

superior colliculus

cerebral aqueduct

oculomotor nucleus

trochlear nucleus

paramedian pontine
reticular formation

superior vestibular
nucleus

fastigial
nucleus

medial longitudinal fasciculus

red nucleus

substantia nigra

medial lemniscus

crus cerebri

reticular nuclei

abducent nucleus

pyramid

accessory olivary
nuclei

inferior olivary
nucleus

lateral
vestibulospinal tract

lateral vestibular
nucleus

nodule

inferior and medial
vestibular nuclei

medial vestibulospinal tract

Figure 10.5   Vestibulocerebellar pathway

2. *Connections of the Spinocerebellum:*

The spinocerebellum receives input as mossy fibers from the spinocerebellar and cuneocerebellar tracts carrying proprioception information relating to position of the limbs. Olivocerebellar fibers terminate as climbing fibers and are considered to be the source of neuronal instructions for complex movements. The spinocerebellum in turn projects to the fastigial nucleus (from the vermis) and to interposed nucleus (from the paravermal cortex). Fibers from the globose and emboliform nuclei terminate in the reticular nuclei, red nucleus and the posterior division of the ventral lateral nucleus of the thalamus. The thalamus in turn projects to the cerebral cortex. Thus, the corticospinal and reticulospinal pathways influence motor neurons to control muscle tone and synergy of muscles (Figure 10.6 and Figure 10.7).

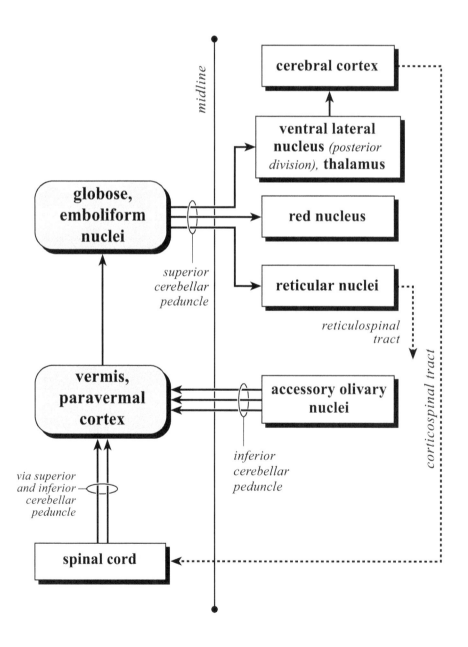

Figure 10.6   Connections of the spinocerebellum

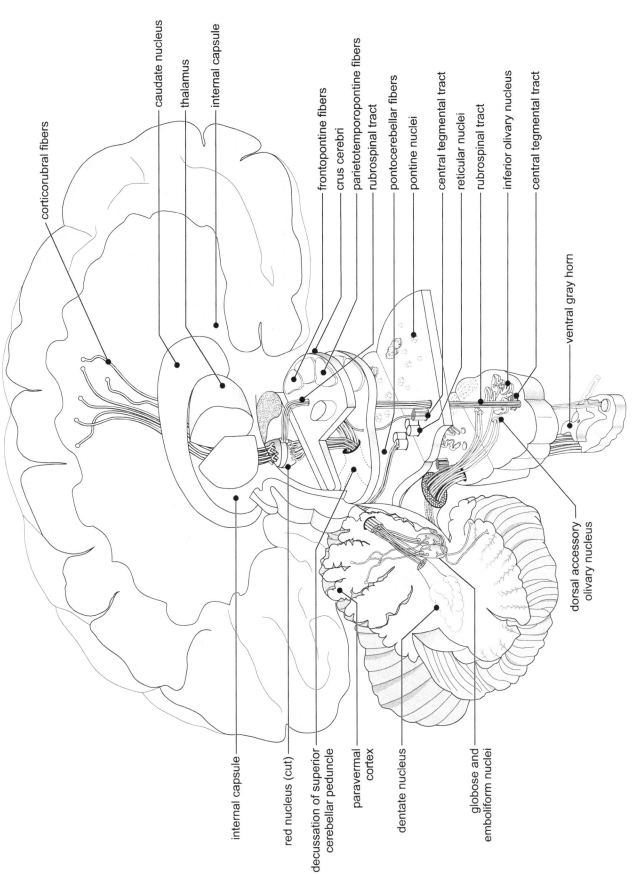

corticorubral fibers

caudate nucleus

thalamus

internal capsule

frontopontine fibers

crus cerebri

parietotemporopontine fibers

rubrospinal tract

pontocerebellar fibers

pontine nuclei

central tegmental tract

reticular nuclei

rubrospinal tract

inferior olivary nucleus

central tegmental tract

ventral gray horn

internal capsule

red nucleus (cut)

decussation of superior
cerebellar peduncle

paravermal
cortex

dentate nucleus

globose and
emboliform nuclei

dorsal accessory
olivary nucleus

Figure 10.7 Spinocerebellar pathway

3. *Connections of the Pontocerebellum:*

The pontocerebellum receives input from the contralateral cerebral cortex. Corticopontine fibers from the ipsilateral cerebral cortex synapse in the pontine nuclei. Axons from the contralateral pontine nuclei form the middle cerebellar peduncle to terminate in the cerebellar hemispheres as mossy fibers. The pontocerebellum projects to the dentate nucleus. Fibers from the dentate nucleus terminate in the contralateral red nucleus and the posterior division of the ventral lateral nucleus of the thalamus. The thalamus in turn projects to the cerebral cortex. Thus, the pontocerebellum via these pathways modifies output from the motor and premotor cortex to ensure smooth coordination of muscles for complex and highly skilled tasks (Figure 10.8 and Figure 10.9).

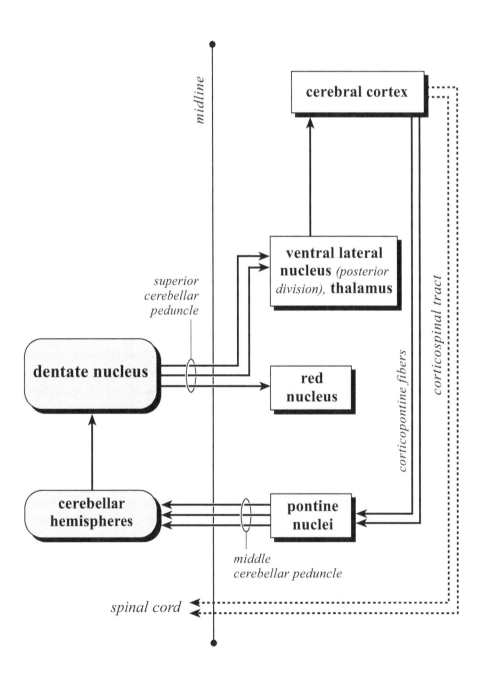

Figure 10.8   Connections of the pontocerebellum

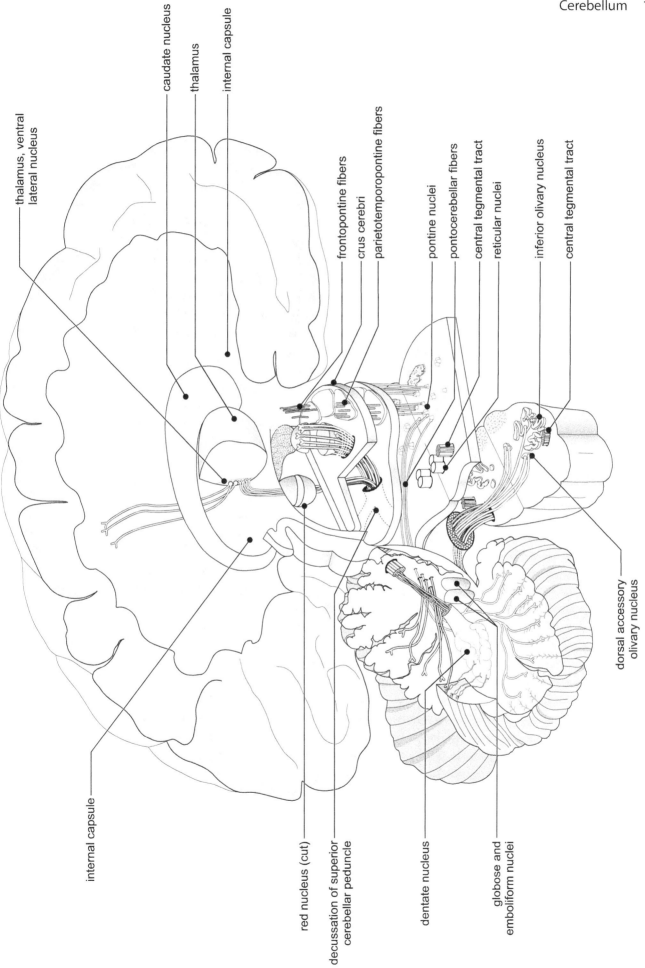

thalamus, ventral lateral nucleus

caudate nucleus

thalamus

internal capsule

frontopontine fibers

crus cerebri

parietotemporopontine fibers

pontine nuclei

pontocerebellar fibers

central tegmental tract

reticular nuclei

inferior olivary nucleus

central tegmental tract

dorsal accessory olivary nucleus

internal capsule

red nucleus (cut)

decussation of superior cerebellar peduncle

dentate nucleus

globose and emboliform nuclei

Figure 10.9   Pontocerebellar pathway

Clinical Notes:

1. *Lesions of the vermis*:
   - commonly occurs in children
   - caused by tumors, such as *medulloblastoma,* in the roof of the fourth ventricle
   - results in loss of coordination of axial muscles and loss of balance, referred to as ***truncal ataxia***. Truncal ataxia is characterized by a lurching gait and a wide-based stance

2. ***Neocerebellar Syndrome:*** involves lesions of the Neocerebellum (Figure 10.10)

   Symptoms are ipsilateral. These are:
   a. ***ataxia*** – loss of coordination of voluntary movements
   b. ***dysmetria*** – hand overshoots or undershoots when attempting to touch a target
   c. ***dysdiadochokinesia*** – inability to perform rapid alternating movements such as pronation and supination.
   d. ***intention tremor*** - tremor during movement, occurs only when a voluntary movement is performed
   e. ***hypotonia*** – decrease muscle tone
   f. ***dysarthria*** – articulation and normal rhythm of speech is impaired due to asynergy of muscles of the tongue, lips and palate

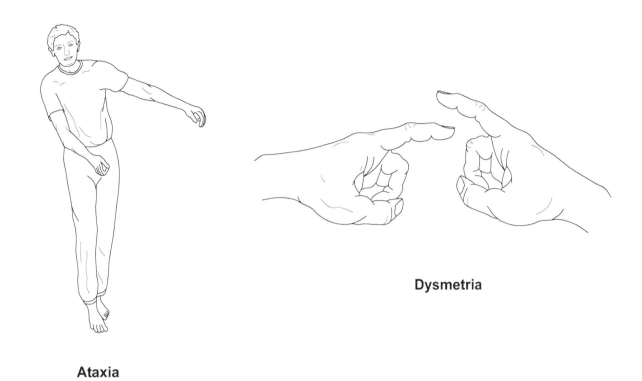

Dysmetria

Ataxia

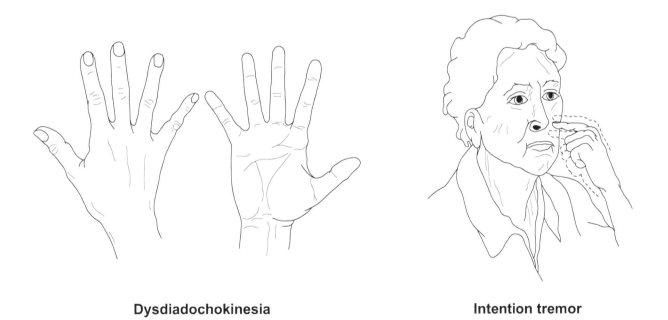

Dysdiadochokinesia

Intention tremor

Figure 10.10   Neocerebellar syndrome

CHAPTER
11

DIENCEPHALON

Overview

The diencephalon is situated between the telencephalon and the midbrain. The two halves of the diencephalon are separated by the third ventricle. The diencephalon contain many groups of nuclei, in addition to many motor, sensory and limbic pathways that relay in the diencephalon before terminating in subcortical structures or the cerebral cortex.

GROSS ANATOMY OF THE DIENCEPHALON:

1. *Location:*

The diencephalon is bounded by the optic chiasm and optic tract and is separated from the midbrain by the mamillary bodies
   a. the medial surface: forms lateral walls of third ventricle.
     • the medial and dorsal surfaces are separated by the ***striae medullaris thalami*** (Figure 13.2)
   b. the dorsal surface: is bounded by the ***fornix***
   c. the ventral surface: is bounded by the ***internal capsule***

2. Components of the Diencephalon:

Consists of the:
   Thalamus: largest component of diencephalon
   Subthalamus: small region, ventral to the thalamus
   Epithalamus: forms dorsal part of the diencephalon
   Hypothalamus: area ventral to the thalamus (Figure 13.2)

I. <u>THALAMUS:</u>

Overview:

The thalamus, the largest component of the diencephalon, is a large oval mass of nuclei that interconnect areas of the cerebral cortex with the basal ganglia, cerebellum and all sensory systems except the olfactory system.

1. Gross Anatomy:

A. *Organization*:

- makes-up 80% of the diencephalon
- large, oval nuclear mass, right and left thalami are fused in the midline of the third ventricle to form the ***intermediate mass*** or massa intermedia (Figure 11.1)
- the *internal medullary lamina*, a Y-shaped sheet of myelinated fibers, subdivides the thalamus into nuclear groups (Figure 11.2), receives input from one or more subcortical structures
- major relay center and source of afferent fibers to the cerebral cortex

B. *Extent and Surfaces* (Figure 13.2):

- Anteriorly: to the interventricular foramen
- Posteriorly: below fornix and corpus callosum
- Inferiorly: hypothalamic sulcus
- Medial surface: lateral walls of 3rd ventricle
- Dorsal surface: fornix and floor of lateral ventricle

2. Thalamic Nuclei:

A. Organization of Thalamic Nuclei:

Refer to Figure 11.2 for the relative positions of the various nuclei

1. ***Anatomical***: the thalamus is subdivided by the internal medullary lamina into eight nuclear groups, named according to their anatomical locations

2. ***Functional***: thalamic nuclei can be classified based on the source of *afferent fibers* and specific pattern of *cortical projections*. Generally, ***specific thalamic nuclei*** project to specific areas of the cerebral cortex; ***association thalamic nuclei*** project to association areas of the cerebral cortex and ***nonspecific thalamic nuclei*** project to wide areas of the cerebral cortex.

A1. Anatomical Organization of Thalamic Nuclei (Figure 11.2):

a. **Anterior Group of Nuclei**: consists of ***one*** nucleus:
- ***Anterior nucleus***: located at the ***anterior tubercle*** of the thalamus and enclosed by the bifurcation of the internal medullary lamina

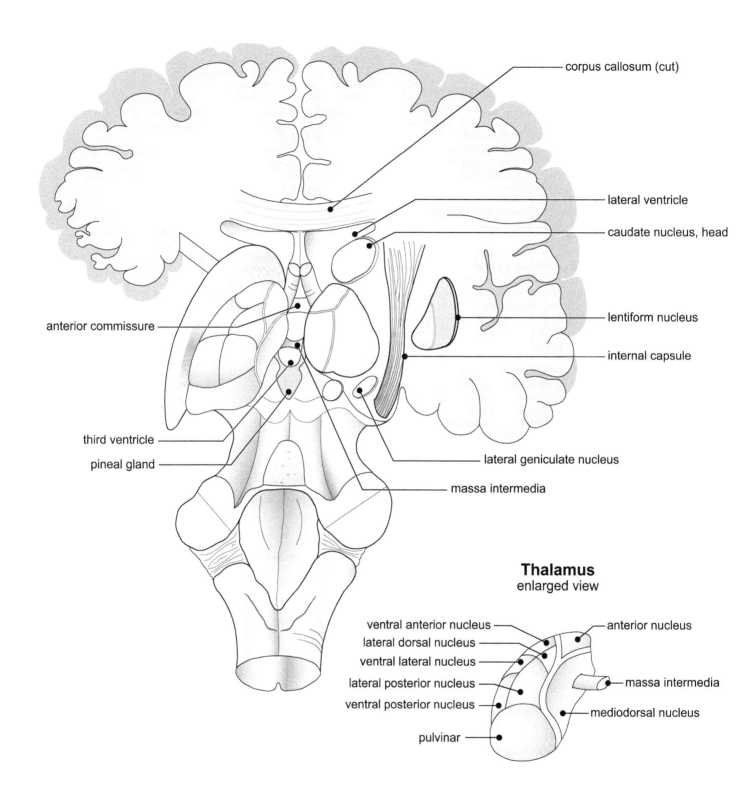

corpus callosum (cut)

lateral ventricle

caudate nucleus, head

anterior commissure

lentiform nucleus

internal capsule

third ventricle

pineal gland

lateral geniculate nucleus

massa intermedia

Thalamus
enlarged view

ventral anterior nucleus

lateral dorsal nucleus

ventral lateral nucleus

lateral posterior nucleus

ventral posterior nucleus

pulvinar

anterior nucleus

massa intermedia

mediodorsal nucleus

Figure 11.1   Dorsal view of the thalamus and epithalamus

b. **Ventral Group of Nuclei**: consists of *five* nuclei arranged anteroposteriorly. These are:
- *Ventral anterior nucleus (VA)*
- *Ventral lateral nucleus* is further subdivided into:
  - ventral lateral, *anterior division* (VLa) and
  - ventral lateral, *posterior division* (VLp)
- *Ventral posterior nucleus* is subdivided into:
  - ventral posterior lateral (VPl)
  - ventral posterior medial (VPm)
- *Medial geniculate nucleus*: is located beneath the pulvinar and lateral to the midbrain
- *Lateral geniculate nucleus*: is located on the lateral part of the posterior limit of the thalamus

c. **Lateral Group of Nuclei**: lies between the internal medullary lamina and the ventral group of nuclei. The lateral group of nuclei consists of *three* nuclei arranged in an anteroposterior sequence as follows:
- *Lateral dorsal nucleus* is located caudal to the anterior nucleus
- *Lateral posterior nucleus*
- *Pulvinar*: largest nucleus of the lateral group of nuclei and forms a prominence on the posterior surface of the thalamus

d. **Medial Group of Nuclei**: consists of *mediodorsal* nucleus and *midline nuclei*:
- *Mediodorsal nucleus*: lies medial to the internal medullary lamina
- *Midline nuclei*: groups of cells associated with the *massa intermedia*

e. **Intralaminar Group of Nuclei**: *small groups* of nuclei contained within the *internal medullary lamina*. These include:
- *Centromedian nucleus*: large, round nucleus located medial to ventral posterior medial nucleus(VPm)
- *Parafascicular nucleus*: located medial to the centromedian nucleus

f. *Additional Nuclei are*:
- *Reticular nucleus*: is a thin layer of cells located lateral to the external medullary lamina

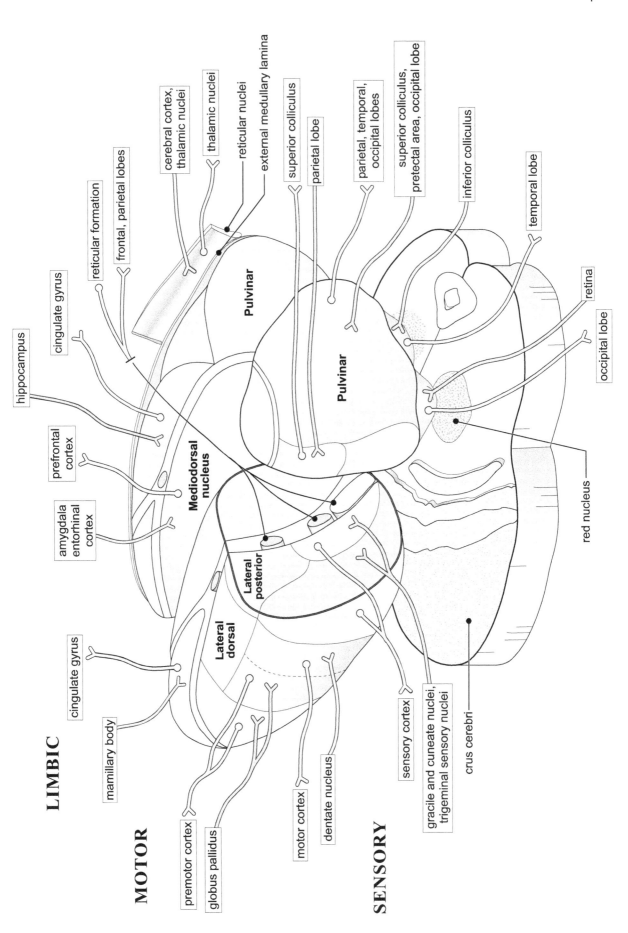

LIMBIC

MOTOR

SENSORY

hippocampus

cingulate gyrus

reticular formation

frontal, parietal lobes

cerebral cortex, thalamic nuclei

thalamic nuclei

reticular nuclei

external medullary lamina

superior colliculus

parietal lobe

parietal, temporal, occipital lobes

superior colliculus, pretectal area, occipital lobe

inferior colliculus

temporal lobe

retina

occipital lobe

prefrontal cortex

amygdala entorhinal cortex

cingulate gyrus

mamillary body

premotor cortex

globus pallidus

motor cortex

dentate nucleus

sensory cortex

gracile and cuneate nuclei, trigeminal sensory nuclei

crus cerebri

red nucleus

Pulvinar

Pulvinar

Mediodorsal nucleus

Lateral posterior

Lateral dorsal

Figure 11.2   Connections of thalamic nuclei

A2. *Functional Organization of Thalamic Nuclei*:

1. **Specific Thalamic Nuclei:** connect to specific *motor* or *sensory areas* of the *cerebral cortex* and include the *ventral group nuclei* and *geniculate nuclei*

   Refer to Table 11.1 and Figure 11.2 for classification, connections and functions of thalamic nuclei.

   Specific thalamic nuclei can be grouped as follows:

   a. **Motor Relay Nuclei** are:

      - *Ventral Anterior nucleus*: relay nucleus for motor planning and behavior
      - *Ventral lateral,anterior division*: relay nucleus for motor planning
      - *Ventral lateral,posterior division*: relay nucleus for motor planning

   b. **Sensory Relay Nuclei**:

      - *Ventral posterior medial nucleus*: involved in somatosensory relay from the *face*
      - *Ventral posterior lateral nucleus*: involved in somatosensory relay from the *body*
      - *Medial geniculate nucleus*: relay nucleus of the *auditory system*
      - *Lateral geniculate nucleus*: relay nucleus of the *visual system*

2. **Association Nuclei**: connect to *frontal* and *parietal-temporal-occipital association cortex*

   The *anterior group, medial group* and *lateral group nuclei* are involved in *sensory integration* and *limbic* and *olfactory* functions.

   Association thalamic nuclei (Table 11.1) can be functionally grouped as follows:

   a. *Limbic and Olfactory Relay Nuclei*:
      - *Anterior nucleus*: relay nucleus of the *limbic* system
      - *Mediodorsal nucleus*: relay nucleus of the *limbic* system
      - *Lateral dorsal nucleus*: relay nucleus of the *limbic* and *olfactory* systems

Table 11.1   Classification, Connections and Functions of Thalamic Nuclei

NUCLEI	FUNCTIONAL CLASSIFICATION	AFFERENTS	EFFERENTS	FUNCTIONS
Ventral anterior	Specific nuclei	Globus pallidus	Frontal lobe; premotor and supplementary motor areas	Motor planning and behavior
Ventral lateral, anterior division	Specific nuclei	Globus pallidus	Premotor; supplementary motor areas	Initiation of movement
Ventral lateral, posterior division	Specific nuclei	Dentate nucleus (contralateral)	Primary motor area	Motor coordination
Ventral posterior lateral	Specific nuclei	Gracile nucleus and cuneate nucleus (contralateral)	Primary somatosensory area	Somatic sensation from contralateral side of body
Ventral posterior medial	Specific nuclei	Trigeminal sensory nuclei (contralateral)	Primary somatosensory area	Somatic sensation from contralateral face and head
Medial geniculate nucleus	Specific nuclei	Inferior colliculus	Primary auditory cortex	Hearing
Lateral geniculate nucleus	Specific nuclei	Ipsilateral halves of retinae	Primary visual cortex	Vision
Anterior group of nuclei	Association nuclei	Mamillary body	Cingulate gyrus	Memory

Table 11.1   Classification, Connections and Functions of Thalamic Nuclei (continued)

NUCLEI	FUNCTIONAL CLASSIFICATION	AFFERENTS	EFFERENTS	FUNCTIONS
Mediodorsal	Association nuclei	Entorhinal cortex, amygdala	Prefrontal cortex	Integrates information with reference to judgement and emotion
Lateral dorsal	Association nuclei	Hippocampus	Cingulate gyrus, visual association cortex	Integration of visual and sensory stimuli
Lateral posterior	Association nuclei	Superior colliculus	Parietal association cortex	Integration of visual and sensory stimuli
Pulvinar	Association nuclei	Pretectal area, visual association cortex	Parietal lobe, frontal cortex, cingulate gyrus	Integration of visual and sensory stimuli
Intralaminar nuclei (centromedian and parafascicular nuclei)	Nonspecific nuclei	Brainstem reticular formation, globus pallidus	Frontal and parietal lobes, striatum	Modulates excitability of cortex in the waking state and arousal from sleep; control of movement
Reticular nucleus	Nonspecific nuclei	Collaterals from corticothalamic and thalamocortical fibers	Thalamic nuclei	Inhibitory regulation of thalamocortical activity

b. ***Sensory Integration Relay Nuclei***:

- ***Lateral posterior nucleus***: relay nucleus for *sensory integration*
- ***Pulvinar:*** relay nucleus for *sensory integration*

3. **Nonspecific Thalamic Nucleus**: connect to widespread areas of the cerebral cortex and can be grouped as follows:

- ***Intralaminar nuclei***: relay nucleus for general information from cortical areas, basal ganglia and brainstem reticular nuclei. These nuclei *modulate activity* of the cortex
- ***Reticular nucleus***: receives and projects within thalamus and is involved in *regulating* thalamocortical activity

Clinical Notes:

Thalamic lesions can affect motor, sensory and mental functions. Symptoms depend on the location and extent of the lesion.

Thalamic syndrome (*Dejerine-Roussy syndrome*): unilateral lesion of the ventral posterior parts of the thalamus. Proprioception, touch and temperature are impaired on the contralateral side of the body. The patient also experiences extreme pain. After a certain threshold, the sensation becomes exaggerated and extremely disagreeable.

II. <u>SUBTHALAMUS</u>

Overview:

The subthalamus is an area inferior to the thalamus and consists of the subthalamic nucleus and tracts that ascend to the thalamus. The subthalamic nucleus is considered to be part of the basal ganglia and is involved in the regulation of movement.

1. Gross Anatomy:

A. *Location:*

- is an area that lies ventral to **thalamus** (Figure 11.3)
- posterolateral to **hypothalamus**
- medial to **internal capsule** and **basis pedunculi**

B. *Organization*:

- consists of the **subthalamic nucleus** and several **somatosensory pathways** (*medial lemniscus, spinothalamic tract and trigeminothalamic tract*) and fiber tracts from the cerebellum and globus pallidus on their way to the thalamus

2. *Nuclei:*

A. **Subthalamic Nucleus**:

- *biconvex* structure (Figure 11.3)
- is anterolateral to the red nucleus
- posterior to basis pedunculi and internal capsule
- has **interconnections** with the **basal ganglia**, and therefore, maintains a **regulatory role** of the basal ganglia in the **control of movement**

3. Connections of the subthalamic nucleus:

A. *Afferents:*

- from **globus pallidus** (external segment) via the **subthalamic fasciculus**

B. *Efferents*:

- excitatory (glutamate) input to the ipsilateral **globus pallidus** *(internal segment)* via the **subthalamic fasciculus** (Figure 12.4) provides a link in an indirect loop through the basal ganglia.
- fibers from the **globus pallidus** (internal segment) travel across the internal capsule as two fiber bundles, the **ansa lenticularis** and the **lenticular fasciculus.** The two bundles join to form the **thalamic fasciculus** to terminate in the ventral lateral (anterior division) of thalamus (Figure 12.3).

Clinical Notes:

Hemiballismus is lesion of the subthalamic nucleus. Damage to the subthalamic nucleus results in decreased excitatory input to the globus pallidus (internal segment), which in turn causes decreased inhibition of the thalamus resulting in unwanted cortical outputs. Lesion of the subthalamic nucleus results in wild, flinging movements of the contralateral upper extremity (Figure 11.4).

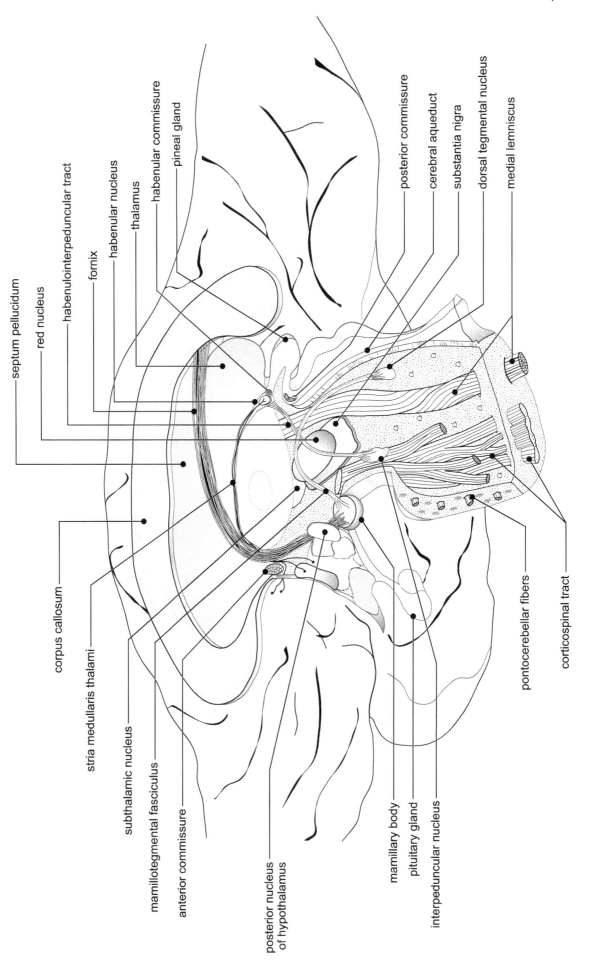

septum pellucidum

red nucleus

habenulointerpeduncular tract

fornix

habenular nucleus

thalamus

habenular commissure

pineal gland

posterior commissure

cerebral aqueduct

substantia nigra

dorsal tegmental nucleus

medial lemniscus

corpus callosum

stria medullaris thalami

subthalamic nucleus

mamillotegmental fasciculus

anterior commissure

posterior nucleus
of hypothalamus

mamillary body

pituitary gland

interpeduncular nucleus

pontocerebellar fibers

corticospinal tract

Figure 11.3 Connections of the subthalamus and epithalamus

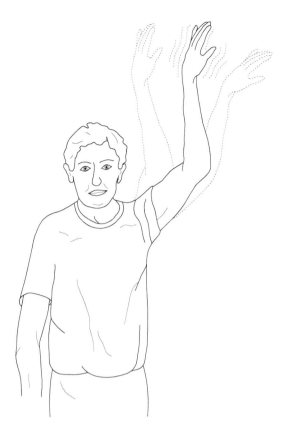

Figure 11.4   Hemiballismus

III. <u>EPITHALAMUS</u>

Overview:

The epithalamus is superior to the thalamus and connects to the hypothalamus and limbic system. It is involved in complex functions such as emotions and behavior.

1. Gross Anatomy:

A. *Location:*

- dorsomedial to the thalamus
- forms the dorsal wall of 3rd ventricle

B. Organization:

- consists of the ***habenular nuclei*** and its ***connections,*** including the ***pineal gland*** (Figure 11.3)

2. Nuclei:

    A. *Habenular Nuclei*:

- superolateral to pineal gland (Figure 11.3)
- consists of the *medial habenular* and *lateral habenular nuclei*
- the habenular nuclei, part of a network that links the *limbic* system, influencing emotion and behavior

    B. *Connections of the habenular nuclei:*

        1. *Afferents*:

- one major *input bundle,* the *stria medullaris thalami,* runs along the dorsomedial border of the thalamus and originates from the:

> septal area (limbic system) ⇒ via *striae medullaris thalami* ⇒ *habenular nuclei* (contralateral).

        2. *Efferents*: *one* major *output bundle,* the *habenulointerpeduncular tract*

- from the *habenular nuclei* to the *interpeduncular nucleus* of the midbrain via the *habenulointerpeduncular tract*
- interconnections of the *interpeduncular nucleus* with the *brainstem reticular nuclei* influence neurons of the *hypothalamus* and the *midbrain reticular formation*

3. PINEAL GLAND

    A. *Anatomy*:

- main structure of the epithalamus (Figure 11.3)
- midline, unpaired structure, shape of a pine cone
- attached to the roof of the third ventricle by the pineal stalk
- consists of pinealocytes, glial cells and capillaries
- pinealocytes synthesize *melatonin* from serotonin

    B. *Functional Significance*:

- melatonin, an antigonadotropic hormone, decreases with the onset of puberty
- secretion of melatonin is decreased with exposure to light, therefore, gonadal function is enhanced with increase in the length of day. Melatonin is said to also have an effect in inducing sleep.
- in animals, it regulates circadian rhythm to light
- in humans, photic stimulation occurs through an indirect route through the hypothalamus

Clinical Notes:
Lesions that destroy pinealocytes are associated with precocious puberty. In contrast, pineal gland tumors delay the onset of puberty.

IV. HYPOTHALAMUS

Overview:

The hypothalamus consists of many nuclei and fiber systems that interconnect components of the central nervous system, autonomic nervous system and the pituitary gland. Accordingly, the hypothalamus is essential to the survival of the individual, controlling temperature regulation, appetite, electrolyte balance, sleep, sexual behavior, including the endocrine functions of the pituitary gland.

1. Gross Anatomy:

A. *Location:*

- forms the floor and lateral walls of the ***third ventricle***
- ventral to ***hypothalamic sulcus***
- bounded by ***optic tracts***, ***optic chiasm*** and ***mamillary bodies***

B. *Organization:*

- divided into ***medial***, **lateral** (or **lateral hypothalamic area**) and **periventricular zones.**
- the *medial zone* is separated from the *lateral zone*, in the parasagittal plane, by the ***fornix*** that traverse the hypothalamus to terminate in the ***mamillary bodies***. The *periventricular zone* is adjacent to the third ventricle
- consists of ***many nuclei*** that connect the ***limbic system***, ***thalamus*** and ***brainstem***.
- connected to the ***pituitary gland*** by the ***hypophyseal stalk*** and ***infundibulum***

2. Regions, Nuclei and Functions:

Details of the specific hypothalamic nuclei will not be covered. The relative positions of the various nuclei are outlined in Figure 11.5

A. **Medial zone***:* consists of three nuclei
B. **Lateral zone**: consists of groups of neurons intermingled with bundles of nerve fibers that form the ***medial forebrain bundle***
C. **Periventricular zone**: contains ***neurons*** that lie beneath the *third ventricle*.

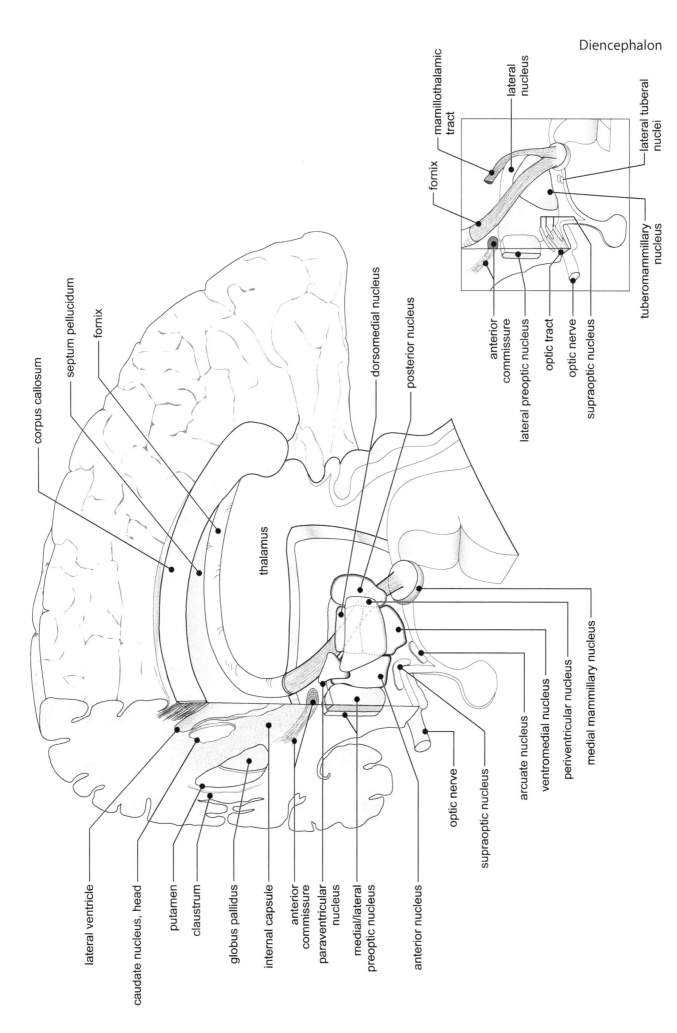

Figure 11.5   Nuclei of the hypothalamus

corpus callosum

septum pellucidum

fornix

thalamus

dorsomedial nucleus

posterior nucleus

fornix

mamillothalamic tract

lateral nucleus

lateral tuberal nuclei

anterior commissure

lateral preoptic nucleus

optic tract

optic nerve

supraoptic nucleus

tuberomammillary nucleus

lateral ventricle

caudate nucleus, head

putamen

claustrum

globus pallidus

internal capsule

anterior commissure

paraventricular nucleus

medial/lateral preoptic nucleus

anterior nucleus

optic nerve

supraoptic nucleus

arcuate nucleus

ventromedial nucleus

periventricular nucleus

medial mammillary nucleus

3. Hypothalamic Afferent and Efferent Fiber Systems:

The hypothalamus connects to various sites and most of these connections are reciprocal. The major areas that the hypothalamus connects with are the limbic system, thalamus, brainstem tegmentum, olfactory system and neocortical areas.

A. **Extrinsic Pathways**:

1. *Afferent fiber systems*:

In general, afferent fibers project to the hypothalamus from the limbic system (hippocampal formation, amygdala and cingulate gyrus), midline thalamic nuclei, brainstem reticular formation, olfactory regions and the frontal cortex. Major afferent fiber systems are summarized in Table 11.2. Refer to Figures 11.6,11.7 and 11.8 and identify the various afferent fiber systems. These are:

i) ***fornix***: projects fibers from the hippocampus to the mamillary bodies and anterior nucleus of the thalamus (Figures 11.6 and 11.7)

ii) ***stria terminalis***: fiber bundle that extends from the amygdaloid nucleus, running in-between the thalamus to nuclei of the hypothalamus

iii) ***stria medullaris thalami***: connects the habenular nuclei with the septal area (limbic system)

iv) ***medial forebrain bundle***: extends throughout the lateral hypothalamus. It contains many diffuse ascending and descending fibers that interconnect the hypothalamus, olfactory cortex, septal area, amygdala and midbrain tegmentum.

v) ***mamillotegmental tract***: fibers from the midbrain reticular formation connect to the mamillary nucleus

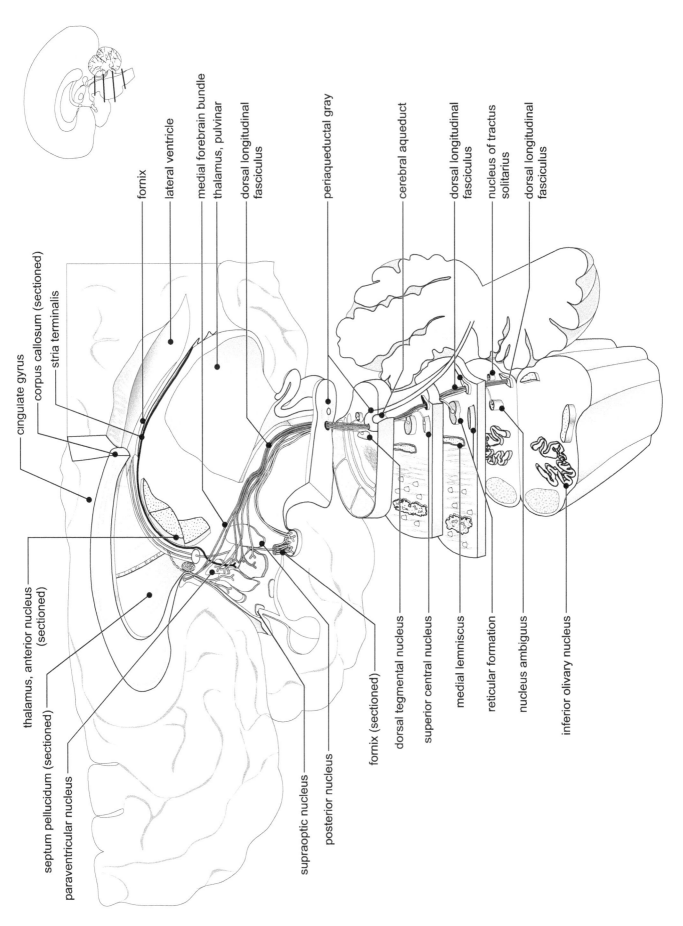

cingulate gyrus

corpus callosum (sectioned)

stria terminalis

fornix

lateral ventricle

medial forebrain bundle

thalamus, pulvinar

dorsal longitudinal fasciculus

periaqueductal gray

cerebral aqueduct

dorsal longitudinal fasciculus

nucleus of tractus solitarius

dorsal longitudinal fasciculus

thalamus, anterior nucleus (sectioned)

septum pellucidum (sectioned)

paraventricular nucleus

supraoptic nucleus

posterior nucleus

fornix (sectioned)

dorsal tegmental nucleus

superior central nucleus

medial lemniscus

reticular formation

nucleus ambiguus

inferior olivary nucleus

Figure 11.6   Afferents and ascending pathways of the hypothalamus

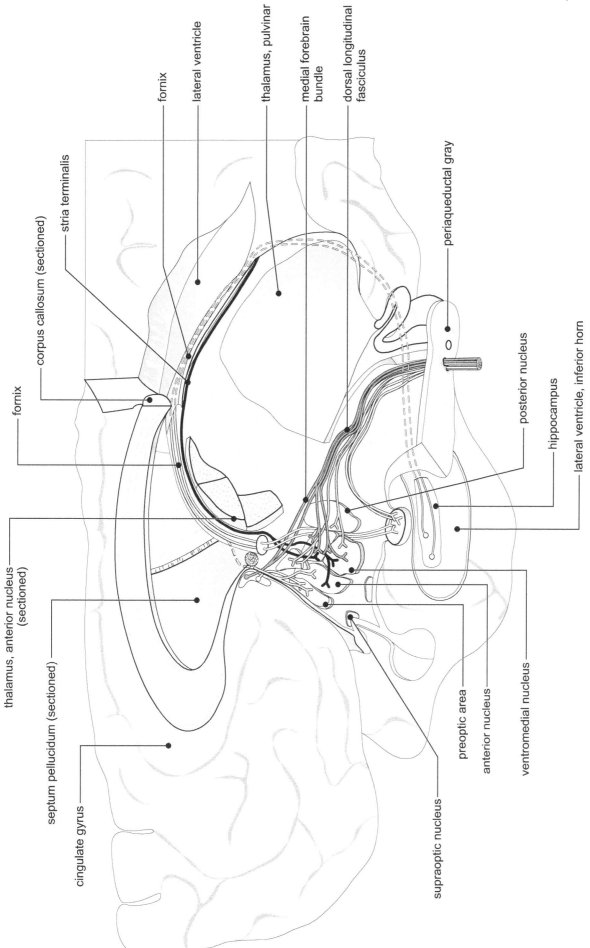

fornix

lateral ventricle

thalamus, pulvinar

medial forebrain bundle

dorsal longitudinal fasciculus

periaqueductal gray

stria terminalis

corpus callosum (sectioned)

fornix

posterior nucleus

hippocampus

lateral ventricle, inferior horn

thalamus, anterior nucleus (sectioned)

septum pellucidum (sectioned)

cingulate gyrus

supraoptic nucleus

preoptic area

anterior nucleus

ventromedial nucleus

Figure 11.7   Afferents of the hypothalamus

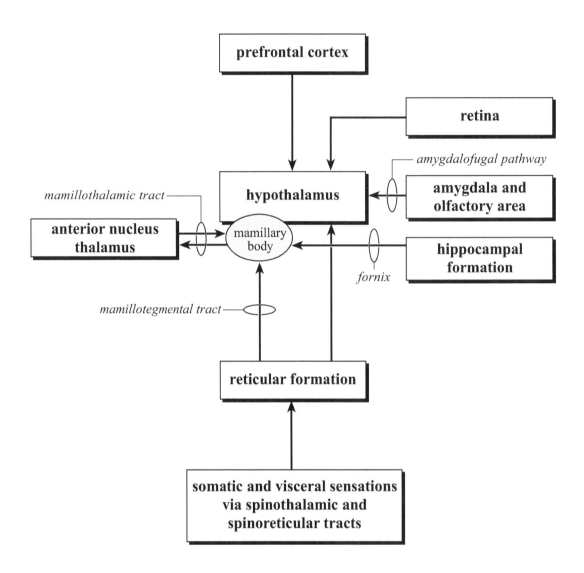

Figure 11.8   Afferent connections of the hypothalamus

Table 11.2   Afferents, Pathways and Functions of the Hypothalamus

ORIGIN	PATHWAY	TERMINATION	FUNCTIONS
Hippocampus, subiculum	*Fornix*	Mamillary body	Receives input from the limbic system and functions in short term memory
Amygdala	*Stria terminalis*	Anterior hypothalamus	Receives input from the limbic system and influences emotional behavior
Olfactory area, septal area,	*Medial forebrain bundle*	Lateral hypothalamus	Links motivation and smell
Periaqueductal gray of midbrain	*Dorsal longitudinal fasciculus*	Medial hypothalamus	Involved in integration of autonomic functions
Reticular formation of brainstem	*Mamillotegmental tract*	Mamillary body	Involved in integration of autonomic functions
Anterior nucleus of thalamus	*Mamillothalamic tract*	Mamillary body	Interconnects hypothalamus and limbic system

2. *Efferent fiber systems*:

The hypothalamus sends fibers to many structures that it receives inputs. Refer to Figures 11.9 to 11.11 and Table 11.3 for a summary of the major efferent pathways:

- i) **fornix**: reciprocal fibers travel in the fornix from the mamillary body to the hippocampal formation
- ii) **mamillothalamic tract**: connects the mamillary bodies with the anterior nucleus of the thalamus, which in turn project to the frontal cortex and cingulate gyrus. These connections comprise a component of the Papez Circuit, which is discussed in Chapter 17
- iii) **mamillotegmental tract**: connects the mamillary body to the midbrain tegmentum and reticular formation
- iv) **medial forebrain bundle**: conveys impulses from the lateral hypothalamus to the septal nuclei and brainstem reticular formation

v) *stria terminalis*: connects hypothalamus with the amygdaloid nucleus
vi) *dorsal longitudinal fasciculus*: extends from the medial hypothalamus to the reticular formation. Descending reticulobulbar and reticulospinal fibers synapse in autonomic cranial nerve nuclei of the brainstem (nucleus ambiguus, dorsal motor nucleus of vagus and solitary nucleus) and autonomic nuclei of the intermediolateral cell column of the spinal cord. Accordingly, the dorsal longitudinal fibers regulates blood pressure, heart rate and digestion.

Table 11.3 Efferents, Pathways and Functions of the Hypothalamus

ORIGIN	PATHWAY	TERMINATION	FUNCTIONS
Mamillary body	*Fornix*	Hippocampal formation	Receives input from the limbic system and functions in short term memory
Hypothalamus (preoptic area)	*Stria terminalis*	Amygdala	Receives input from the limbic system and influences reproductive behavior
Lateral hypothalamus	*Medial forebrain bundle*	septal area, brainstem reticular formation	Plays a role in motivation
Hypothalamus	*Dorsal longitudinal fasciculus*	Reticular formation	Involved in autonomic responses
Mamillary body	*Mamillothalamic tract*	Anterior nucleus of thalamus	Interconnects hypothalamus and limbic system
Paraventricular nucleus, lateral hypothalamic area and posterior hypothalamus	*Descending autonomic fibers*	Autonomic and cranial nuclei, spinal motor neurons	Influences cardiovascular and endocrine responses
Anterior and posterior hypothalamus	*Hypothalamic-prefrontal tract*	Prefrontal cortex	Links autonomic responses to emotion
Hypothalamus	*Hypothalamo-hypophyseal tract*	Pituitary gland	Hormones synthesized are released in the neurohypophysis

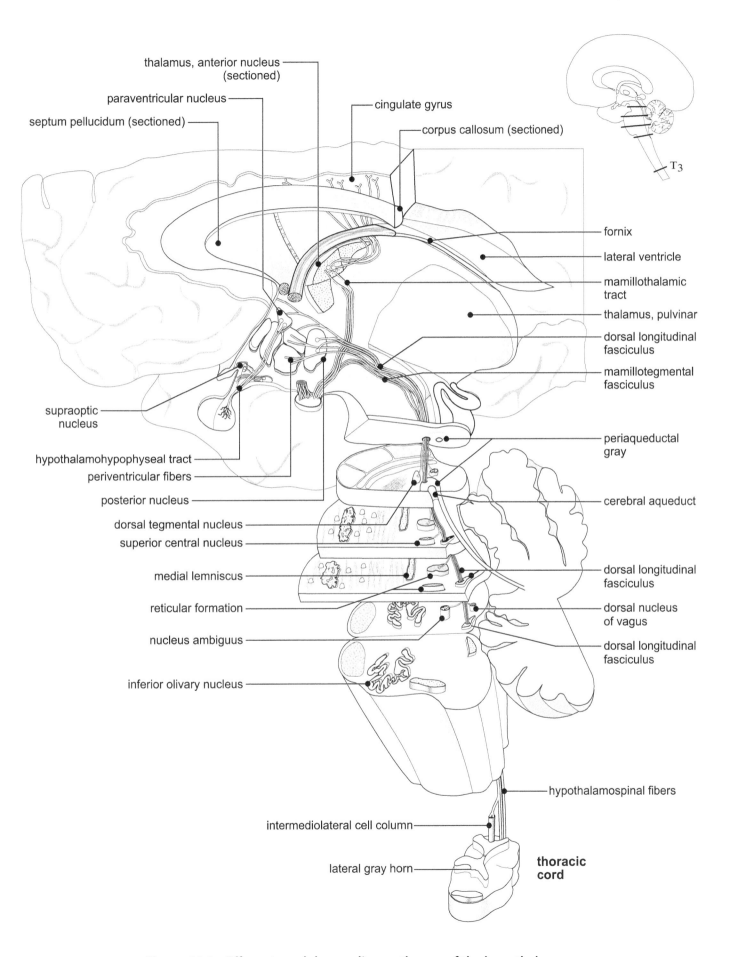

thalamus, anterior nucleus
(sectioned)

paraventricular nucleus

septum pellucidum (sectioned)

cingulate gyrus

corpus callosum (sectioned)

T₃

fornix

lateral ventricle

mamillothalamic
tract

thalamus, pulvinar

dorsal longitudinal
fasciculus

mamillotegmental
fasciculus

supraoptic
nucleus

periaqueductal
gray

hypothalamohypophyseal tract

periventricular fibers

posterior nucleus

cerebral aqueduct

dorsal tegmental nucleus

superior central nucleus

medial lemniscus

dorsal longitudinal
fasciculus

reticular formation

dorsal nucleus
of vagus

nucleus ambiguus

dorsal longitudinal
fasciculus

inferior olivary nucleus

hypothalamospinal fibers

intermediolateral cell column

**thoracic
cord**

lateral gray horn

Figure 11.9   Efferents and descending pathways of the hypothalamus

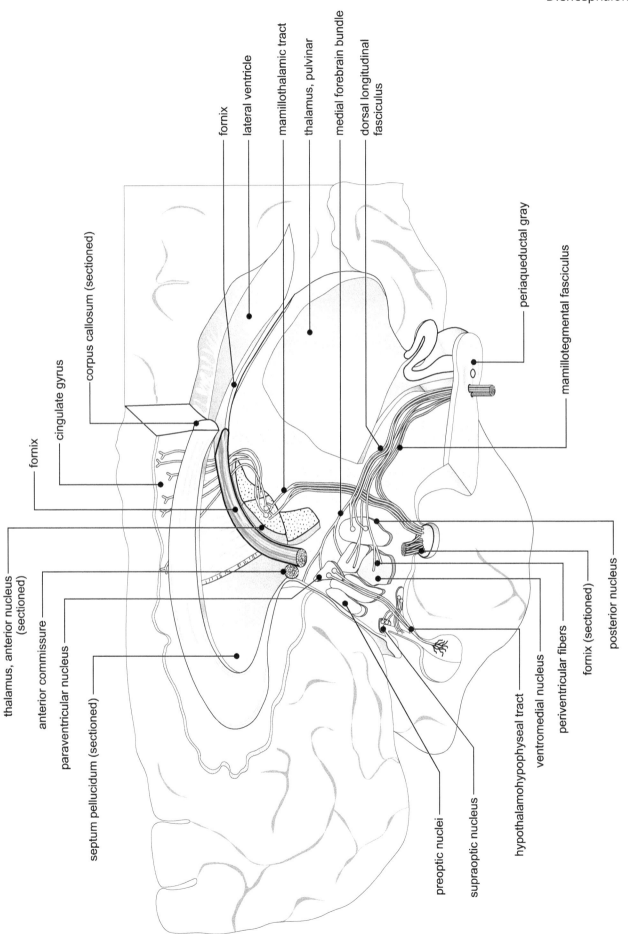

fornix

lateral ventricle

mamillothalamic tract

thalamus, pulvinar

medial forebrain bundle

dorsal longitudinal fasciculus

periaqueductal gray

mamillotegmental fasciculus

corpus callosum (sectioned)

cingulate gyrus

fornix

thalamus, anterior nucleus (sectioned)

anterior commissure

paraventricular nucleus

septum pellucidum (sectioned)

preoptic nuclei

supraoptic nucleus

hypothalamohypophyseal tract

ventromedial nucleus

periventricular fibers

fornix (sectioned)

posterior nucleus

Figure 11.10   Efferents of the hypothalamus

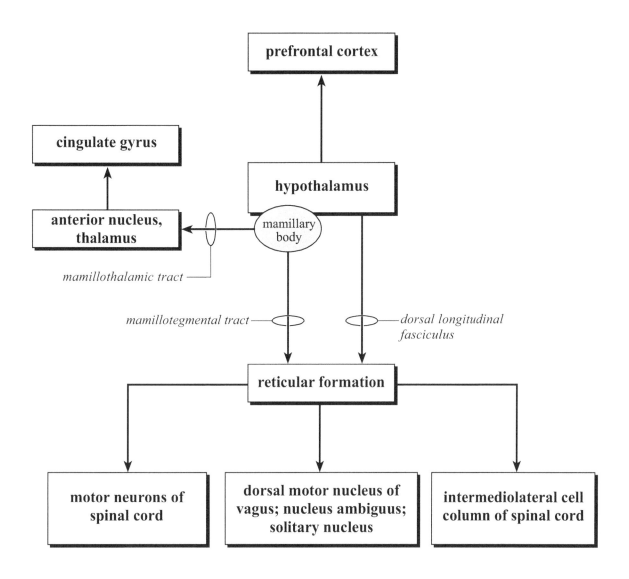

Figure 11.11   Efferent connections of the hypothalamus

B. **Intrinsic Connections**:

1. **Autonomic Functions:**

   a. **Anterior hypothalamus** is involved in the following functions:

      i. **Parasympathetic function:**
         • decreases heart rate, blood pressure, increases functions of the gastrointestinal tract

      ii. promotes heat loss such as vasodilation and sweating

b. **Posterior hypothalamus** is involved in the following functions:

    i. **Sympathetic:**
- increases heart rate, blood pressure, decrease in gastrointestinal functions

    ii. promotes conservation and production of heat such as vasoconstriction and shivering

c. *Lateral zone of the hypothalamus:*
- is the 'hunger' or 'feeding' center
- neurons of the lateral hypothalamic synthesize orexins, which are neuropeptides that regulate food intake and the sleep-wake cycle

d. *Ventromedial nuclei of the hypothalamus:*
- is the 'satiety' center

Clinical Notes:

Lesions of the hypothalamus involves many different disorders and only a few examples will be described. A lesion of the anterior hypothalamus will result in hyperthermia and disruption of the parasympathetic functions. A lesion of the posterior hypothalamus results in hypothermia and disruption of the sympathetic functions. A lesion of the lateral hypothalamus results in loss of appetite and a decrease in body weight. A lesion of the ventromedial nucleus of the hypothalamus results in overeating and obesity

2. **Neuroendocrine Functions:**

a. **Anterior pituitary:**

- hormones are released through a system of blood vessels, the ***hypothalamic-hypophyseal portal system***. *Releasing* or *Inhibiting hormones* synthesized in the hypothalamus stimulates or inhibits release of hormones secreted by the anterior pituitary. In turn, the anterior pituitary controls most of the endocrine glands and influences many processes such as reproduction and metabolism.

b. *Posterior pituitary:*

- hormones secreted by the *supraoptic* and *paraventricular nuclei* of the hypothalamus and released in the posterior pituitary are ***oxytocin*** and ***vasopressin.***

CHAPTER
12

CORPUS STRIATUM

Overview

The corpus striatum consists of a group of nuclei located in the white matter of the cerebrum. The corpus striatum forms part of a group of interconnected nuclei that are involved in motor function and collectively referred to as the *basal ganglia*. Functionally, the basal ganglia consists of the corpus striatum, subthalamic nucleus and the substantia nigra. The corpus striatum, in turn consists of the caudate nucleus and the lentiform nucleus.

I. Corpus Striatum

A. *Components:*

Consists of the following as indicated in Figure 12.1:

i. *caudate nucleus*

- is C-shaped and located medially, in the wall of the lateral ventricle
- it consists of a **head** and a slender *tail*. The head bulges into the anterior horn of the lateral ventricle while the tail extends into the temporal lobe of the cerebrum. The tail of the caudate nucleus is continuous with the amygdala

ii. *lentiform nucleus*

- is wedge shaped and located laterally
- it consists of a lateral portion, the *putamen* and a medial portion, the **globus pallidus**
- the globus pallidus in turn is divided into an *external* (*lateral*) *segment* and an *internal* (*medial*) *segment*.

B. Traditional Concepts:

Corpus Striatum = caudate nucleus + lentiform nucleus
Neostriatum or **striatum** = caudate nucleus + putamen

Pallidum = globus pallidus
Basal ganglia = *corpus striatum*, *substantia nigra* and *subthalamic nucleus*

C. Spatial relations of Corpus striatum to the internal capsule:

Figure 12.2 is a schematic diagram of the corpus striatum, viewed from above. The left cerebral hemisphere has been sectioned to show the relationship of the corpus striatum to the *anterior* and *posterior limbs* and *genu* of the *internal capsule*. The right hemisphere is sectioned at a higher level to show the caudate nucleus arching backwards and extending into the inferior horn of the lateral ventricle.   The spatial relations are as follows:

- medial to the anterior limb is the caudate nucleus
- medial to the posterior limb is the thalamus
- lateral to the anterior and posterior limbs are the globus pallidus and putamen
- lateral to the genu is the lentiform nucleus
- located lateral to the lentiform nucleus is the *external capsule*, *claustrum*, *extreme capsule* and *insula* (Figure 15.1)

D. Connections of the Corpus striatum:

Refer to Figure 12.3 for the following connections.

1. **Neostriatum**

   a. *Afferents*:

   - *corticostriate fibers* originate from the association cortex   ⇒ caudate nucleus and from the motor and sensory cortex   ⇒ putamen. Glutamate is the neurotransmitter
   - *thalamostriate fibers* - from the intralaminar nuclei of the thalamus
   - *nigrostriate fibers* - from pars compacta of substantia nigra Dopamine is the neurotransmitter

   b. *Efferents*:

   - *striatopallidal fibers* from the striatum   ⇒   globus pallidus
   - *striatonigral fibers* from the striatum   ⇒   substantia nigra (pars reticulata)

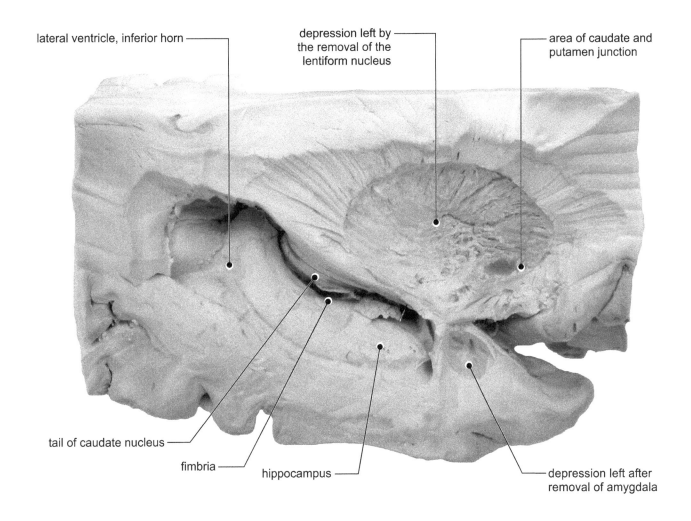

lateral ventricle, inferior horn

depression left by
the removal of the
lentiform nucleus

area of caudate and
putamen junction

tail of caudate nucleus

fimbria

hippocampus

depression left after
removal of amygdala

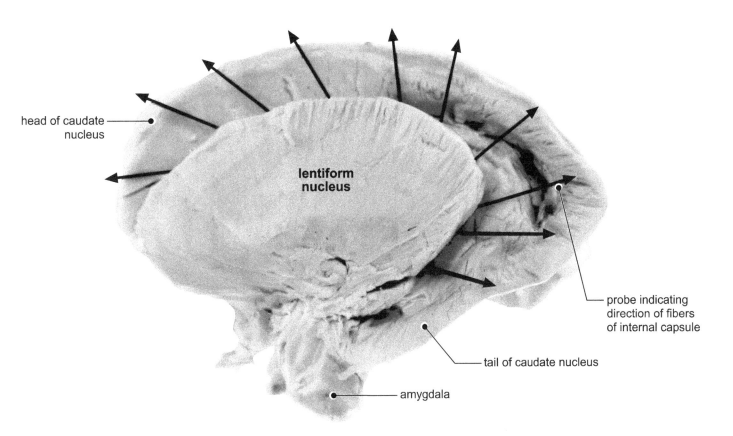

head of caudate
nucleus

lentiform
nucleus

probe indicating
direction of fibers
of internal capsule

tail of caudate nucleus

amygdala

Figure 12.1   Dissection of the corpus striatum

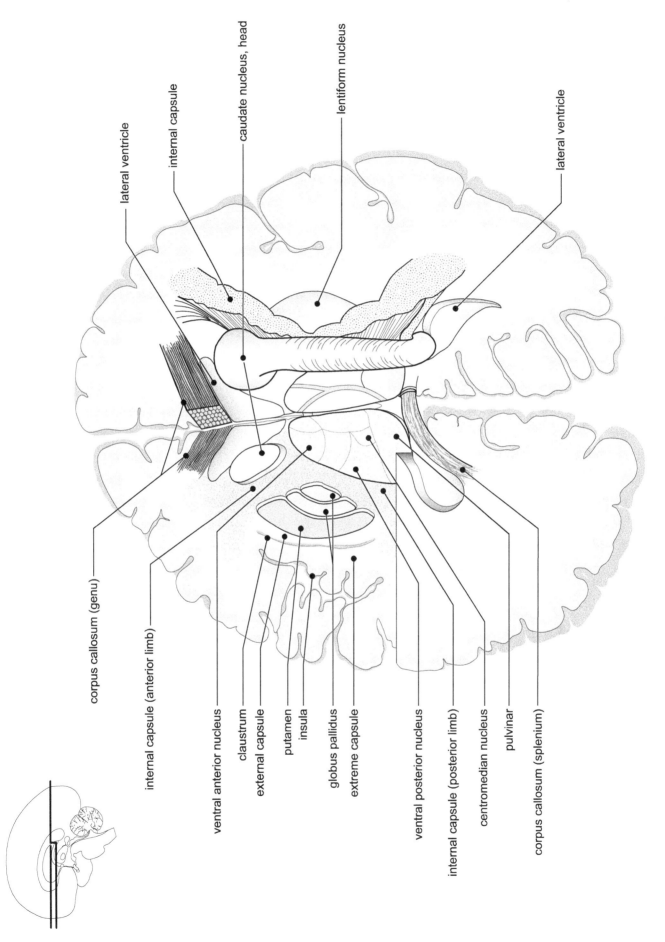

lateral ventricle

internal capsule

caudate nucleus, head

lentiform nucleus

lateral ventricle

corpus callosum (genu)

internal capsule (anterior limb)

ventral anterior nucleus

claustrum

external capsule

putamen

insula

globus pallidus

extreme capsule

ventral posterior nucleus

internal capsule (posterior limb)

centromedian nucleus

pulvinar

corpus callosum (splenium)

Figure 12.2   Corpus striatum and internal capsule

2. **Paleostriatum**

    a. *Afferents*:

- *striatopallidal fibers* from the striatum ⇒ globus pallidus
- *subthalamic fasciculus* from the subthalamic nucleus ⇒ globus pallidus (internal segment)

    b. *Efferents*:

- *pallidothalamic fibers*: takes two routes from the internal segment of the globus pallidus. These are:
  - i. fibers cross the internal capsule as the *lenticular fasciculus*
  - ii. fibers curve around the internal capsule as the *ansa lenticularis*

  These two fasciculi join to form the *thalamic fasciculus*, which terminates in the *ventral anterior* and *ventral lateral (anterior division) nuclei* of the thalamus
- *subthalamic fasciculus* connects subthalamic nucleus and the external segment of the globus pallidus

II. Connections of the Basal ganglia:

The flow of information through the basal ganglia is illustrated in Figure 12.4. Generally, there are two loops, a *direct loop* and an *indirect loop*, from the striatum to the thalamus. Nigrostriate fibers excite D1 receptors of striatal neurons of the direct loop and inhibit D2 receptors of striatal neurons of the indirect loop

In the *direct loop (GABA-substance P)*, the pathway is as follows:

cortical fibers are excitatory to the neostriatum ⇒ inhibitory to internal pallidum and substantia nigra (pars reticulata) ⇒ resulting in decreased inhibition of thalamus ⇒ thalamocortical projections are excitatory to the premotor and supplementary motor areas of the cortex ⇒ movements are facilitated

In the *Indirect loop (GABA-enkephalin)*, the pathway is as follows:

cortical fibers are excitatory to the neostriatum ⇒ inhibitory to the external pallidum ⇒ resulting in decreased inhibition of the subthalamic nucleus ⇒ increased excitation of internal pallidum ⇒ resulting in increased inhibition of thalamus ⇒ decreased excitation of premotor and supplementary motor areas of the cortex ⇒ movements are inhibited

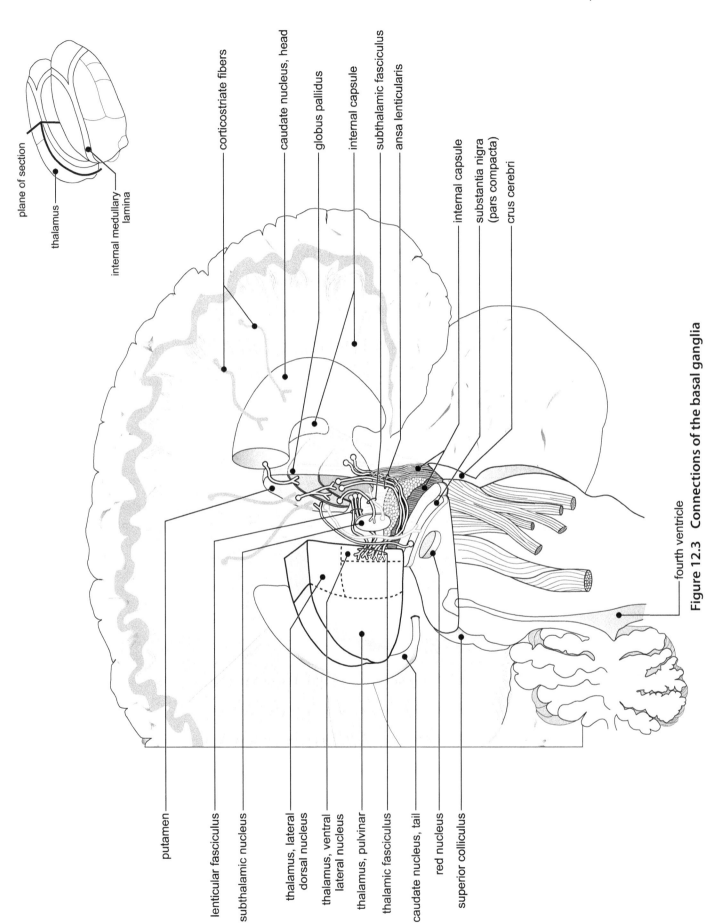

plane of section

thalamus

internal medullary lamina

corticostriate fibers

caudate nucleus, head

globus pallidus

internal capsule

subthalamic fasciculus

ansa lenticularis

internal capsule

substantia nigra (pars compacta)

crus cerebri

fourth ventricle

putamen

lenticular fasciculus

subthalamic nucleus

thalamus, lateral dorsal nucleus

thalamus, ventral lateral nucleus

thalamus, pulvinar

thalamic fasciculus

caudate nucleus, tail

red nucleus

superior colliculus

Figure 12.3   Connections of the basal ganglia

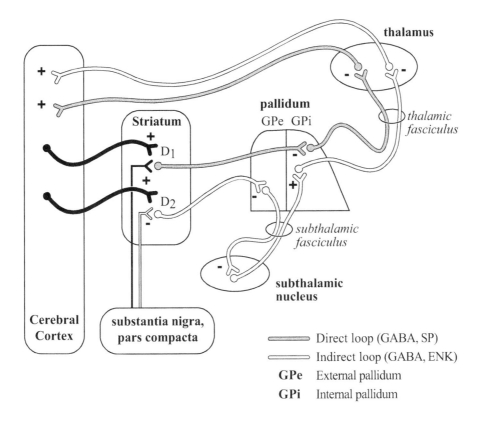

Figure 12.4   Neuronal circuitry of the direct and indirect loops of the basal ganglia

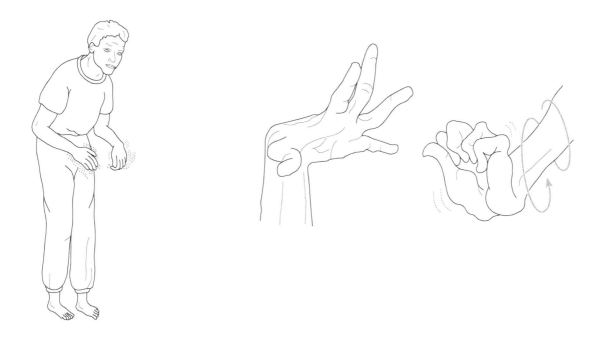

Parkinson's   **Athetosis and Chorea**

Figure 12.5   Basal ganglia disorders

Clinical Notes:

Lesions of the basal ganglia results in disorderly, involuntary movements referred to as *dyskinesias*, and may be classified as hypokinetic disorders or hyperkinetic disorders. Hyperkinetic disorders are displayed as chorea, athetosis or ballism.

i.   ***Chorea*** are rapid movements of face, trunk and limbs
   •   these movements often resemble fragments of normal voluntary movements. example: ***Huntington's chorea***
   •   lesion involves the caudate nucleus
   •   is an inherited disorder
   •   onset: usually 40-50 years

ii. ***Hemiballismus***:
   •   lesion involves the subthalamic nucleus
   •   manifested by large flinging movements of the upper extremities

iii. ***Athetosis*** (without position)
   •   lesion involves the external segment of the globus pallidus
   •   are slow; twisting involuntary movements of the extremities

iv. ***Parkinson's disease***
   •   lesion involves the substantia nigra, pars compacta
   •   symptoms are resting tremor, bradykinesia and rigidity

v.   ***Wilson's disease***
   •   lesion involves the putamen and is caused by an inherited disorder associated with an error in copper metabolism
   •   symptoms involve tremor, muscular rigidity and dystonia

CHAPTER
13

THE CEREBRAL HEMISPHERES

Overview

The cerebrum is the largest portion of the brain. It consists of the right and left cerebral hemispheres that are separated by the longitudinal cerebral fissure and are connected internally by the corpus callosum. The outer gray matter is the cerebral cortex, beneath the cortex is the cerebral white matter which contains tracts and nuclei. The cortex is irregularly convoluted forming gyri, that are separated by fissures or sulci. Major sulci divide the cerebral hemispheres into four lobes that are named according to the skull bones that overlie them. Each cerebral hemisphere contain the lateral ventricles, which contain cerebrospinal fluid.

1. *Gross Anatomy:*

A. *Major Sulci and fissures:*

The major sulci divide the cerebral hemisphere into the *frontal*, *parietal*, *insular*, *temporal* and *occipital lobes*. The *frontal poles* of the hemisphere project into the anterior cranial fossa, the *occipital poles* project posteriorly into the posterior cranial fossa and the *temporal poles* project inferiorly into the middle cranial fossa.

Only the major sulci and gyri will be covered in this chapter.

The major sulci (Figure 13.1) are:

   i.   *central sulcus*:
   - on the lateral surface of the cerebrum
   - begins at the superior border, about 1cm posterior to the midpoint between the frontal and occipital poles of the hemisphere
   - it separates the frontal and parietal lobes

   ii. **lateral sulcus:**
   - begins on the inferior surface and extends laterally between the frontal and temporal lobes, dividing into three rami. These are the *posterior ramus,* the *anterior ramus* and *ascending ramus*
   - at the bottom of the lateral sulcus is the *insula*
   - the lateral sulcus separates the frontal and parietal lobes from the temporal lobe

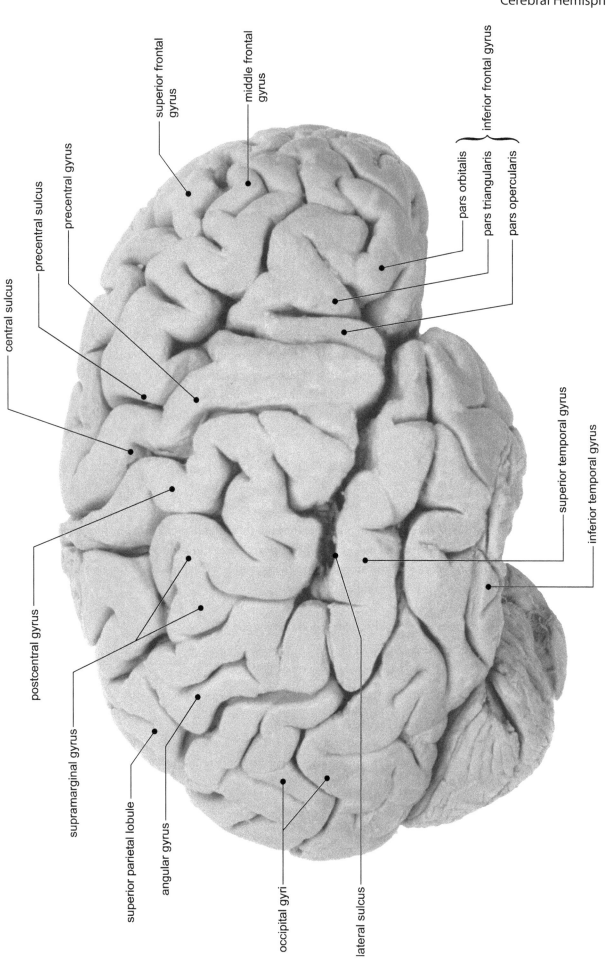

superior frontal gyrus

middle frontal gyrus

inferior frontal gyrus

pars orbitalis

pars triangularis

pars opercularis

precentral sulcus

precentral gyrus

central sulcus

superior temporal gyrus

inferior temporal gyrus

postcentral gyrus

supramarginal gyrus

superior parietal lobule

angular gyrus

occipital gyri

lateral sulcus

Figure 13.1   Lateral surface of the right cerebral hemisphere

iii. *calcarine sulcus*:
- located on the medial surface of the occipital lobe (Figure 13.2)
- it extends from below the posterior end of the corpus callosum to the occipital pole

iv. *parieto-occipital sulcus*:
- on the medial surface, extending from the calcarine sulcus to the superior border of the hemisphere
- separates the occipital and parietal lobes

v. *longitudinal cerebral fissure*:
- separates the two cerebral hemispheres

B. Lobes of the Cerebral Hemispheres:

Each cerebral hemisphere has *lateral*, *medial* and *inferior surfaces* (Figures 13.1 to 13.3).. The four major lobes of the hemisphere are:

i. *Frontal lobe*:
- is located anterior to the central sulcus and above the lateral sulcus.

On its *lateral surface* (Figure 13.1) are the:
- *precentral gyrus*, anterior to the central sulcus and limited anteriorly by the *precentral sulcus*.
- anterior to the precentral sulcus, the frontal lobe can be subdivided into the *superior frontal gyrus*, *middle frontal gyrus* and *inferior frontal gyrus*
- the inferior frontal gyrus is demarcated by the anterior and ascending rami of the lateral sulcus into the *opercular*, *triangular* and *orbital parts* (Figure 13.1).

On its *medial surface* (Figure 13.2) are the:
- *cingulate sulcus* is located above the cingulate gyrus
- *cingulate gyrus* is located immediately above the corpus callosum
- the anterior part of the *paracentral lobule* is the continuation of the precentral gyrus
- *subcallosal gyrus* (*septal area*) is located below the rostrum of the corpus callosum

On its *inferior surface* (Figure 13.3) are the:
- *orbitofrontal cortex, olfactory bulb and olfactory tract*. The olfactory tract terminates at the *olfactory trigone*, which abuts the *anterior perforated substance*

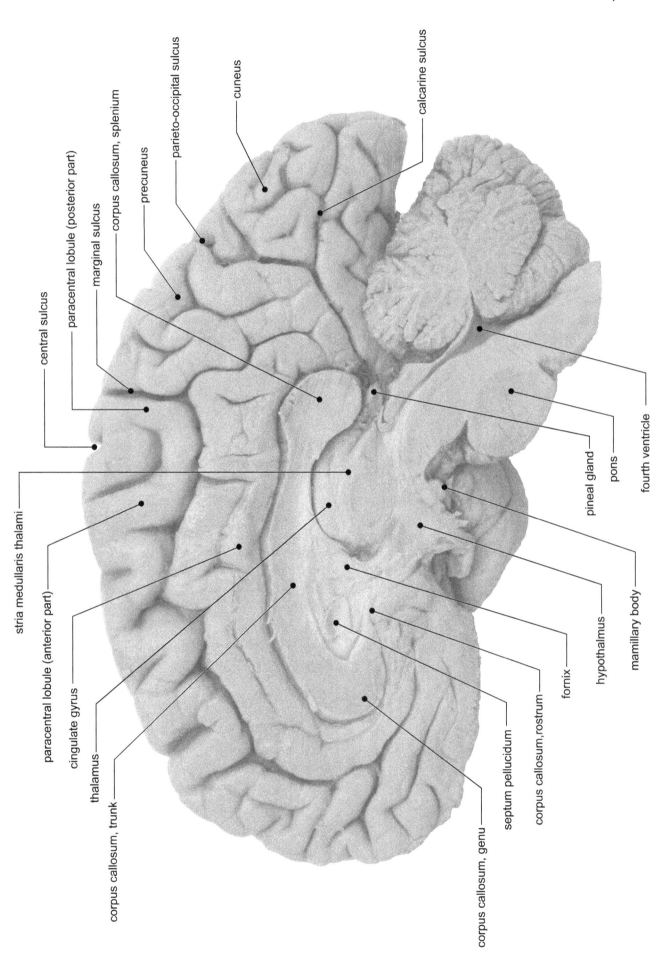

cuneus

calcarine sulcus

parieto-occipital sulcus

precuneus

corpus callosum, splenium

marginal sulcus

paracentral lobule (posterior part)

central sulcus

stria medullaris thalami

paracentral lobule (anterior part)

cingulate gyrus

thalamus

corpus callosum, trunk

corpus callosum, genu

septum pellucidum

corpus callosum, rostrum

fornix

hypothalmus

mamillary body

fourth ventricle

pons

pineal gland

Figure 13.2   Sagittal section of the right cerebral hemisphere

ii. *Parietal lobe*:
- is located between the central sulcus and parieto-occipital sulcus

On its *lateral surface* (Figure 13.1) are the:
- *postcentral gyrus*, posterior to the central sulcus
- posterior to the postcentral gyrus, the parietal lobe can be subdivided into the *superior parietal lobule* and *inferior parietal lobule.*
- the areas of the inferior parietal lobule that surround the posterior ends of the superior temporal sulcus and the lateral sulcus are the *angular* and *supramarginal gyri*, respectively.

On its *medial surface* (Figure 13.2) are the:
- posterior part of the *paracentral lobule*, a continuation of the postcentral gyrus
- *precuneus*, posterior to the paracentral lobule and continuous with the superior parietal lobule

iii. *Insular lobe (Insula)*:
- is located deep within the lateral sulcus and concealed by the frontal, temporal and parietal lobes
- the insula is outlined by the *circular sulcus*
- inferior part of the insula is the *limen insulae*

iv. *Temporal lobe*:
- separated from the frontal and parietal lobes by the lateral sulcus

On its *lateral surface* (Figure 13.1) are the:
- *superior temporal gyrus*, *middle temporal gyrus* and *inferior temporal gyrus* separated by the *superior temporal* and *inferior temporal sulci*
- the superior temporal gyrus forms the floor of the lateral sulcus.
- the anterior part of the superior temporal gyrus is marked by the *transverse temporal gyri* (*Heschl's convolutions*)
- the posterosuperior part of the superior temporal gyrus is the *planum temporale*

On its *inferior surface* (Figure 13.3) are the:
- *parahippocampal gyrus* and *lateral occipitotemporal gyri*
- the anterior most extent of the *parahippocampal gyrus* is the *uncus*
- the *parahippocampal gyrus* is continuous with the cingulate gyrus at the area of the splenium of the corpus callosum

v. *Occipital lobe*:
- extends from the parieto-occipital sulcus and the occipital pole

On its *medial surface* (Figure 13.2) are the:
- *cuneus,* located between the parieto-occipital and calcarine sulcus

On its *inferior surface* is the:
- *medial occipitotemporal gyrus,* located along the lateral side of the parahippocampal gyrus

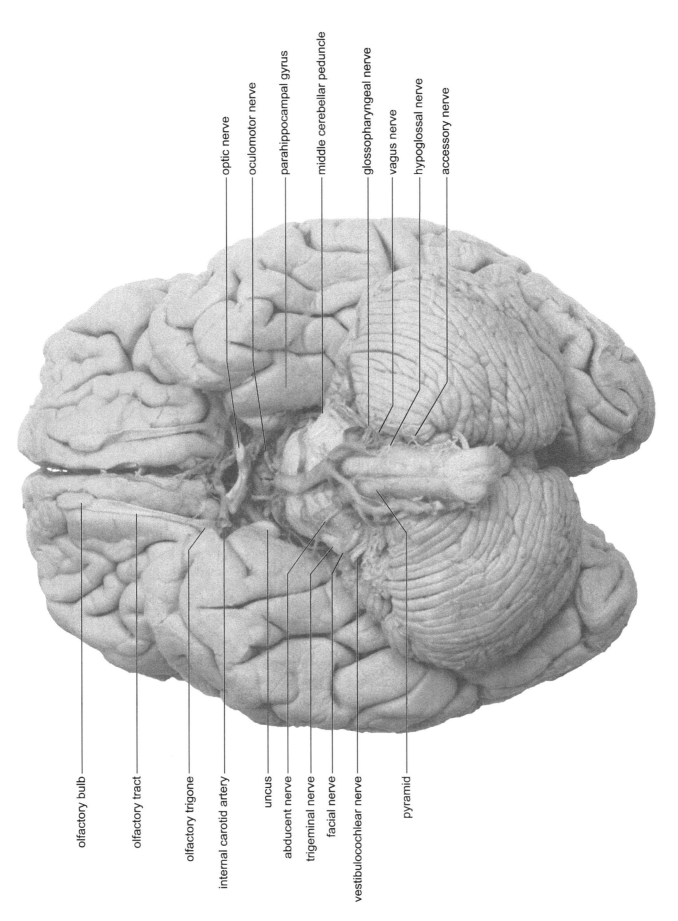

olfactory bulb

olfactory tract

olfactory trigone

internal carotid artery

uncus

abducent nerve

trigeminal nerve

facial nerve

vestibulocochlear nerve

pyramid

optic nerve

oculomotor nerve

parahippocampal gyrus

middle cerebellar peduncle

glossopharyngeal nerve

vagus nerve

hypoglossal nerve

accessory nerve

Figure 13.3   Inferior surface of the brain

CHAPTER
14

HISTOLOGY AND FUNCTIONAL LOCALIZATION OF THE CEREBRAL CORTEX

Overview

The cerebral cortex, the outer gray matter, consists of cell bodies of neurons, axons and dendrites that are arranged distinctly in different regions of the gray matter. The cortex contains of about 10 to 20 billion neurons that are grouped into functional units of columns or modules. Each module responds to a specific type of stimulus. On the basis of its cytoarchitecture, specific functions have been charted for each area of the cerebral cortex. The cerebral cortex is the center of the brain, it perceives sensations, controls skilled movements and is necessary for language, memory and higher mental functions

1. Organization:

Based on the number of cell layers, the cerebral cortex can be classified as consisting of the following:

Paleocortex: includes the rhinencephalon (olfactory cortex)
Archicortex: includes the hippocampal formation
Neocortex: is most recent in evolution and consists of six layers

2. Histology of the Cerebral Cortex:

a. The gray matter consists of the following cell types as indicated in Figure 14.1:

    i. *pyramidal cells*:
- are the principal cells of the cortex, found in all but the outermost layer of the cortex
- consists of apical and laterally directed dendrites, toward the cortical surface
- giant pyramidal cells (Betz cells) are present in the primary motor area (precentral gyrus)
- axon arises from the base of the cell body and enters the white matter as efferents; are excitatory and utilize glutamate as the neurotransmitter

    ii. *fusiform cells*:
- are located in the deepest layer of the cortex

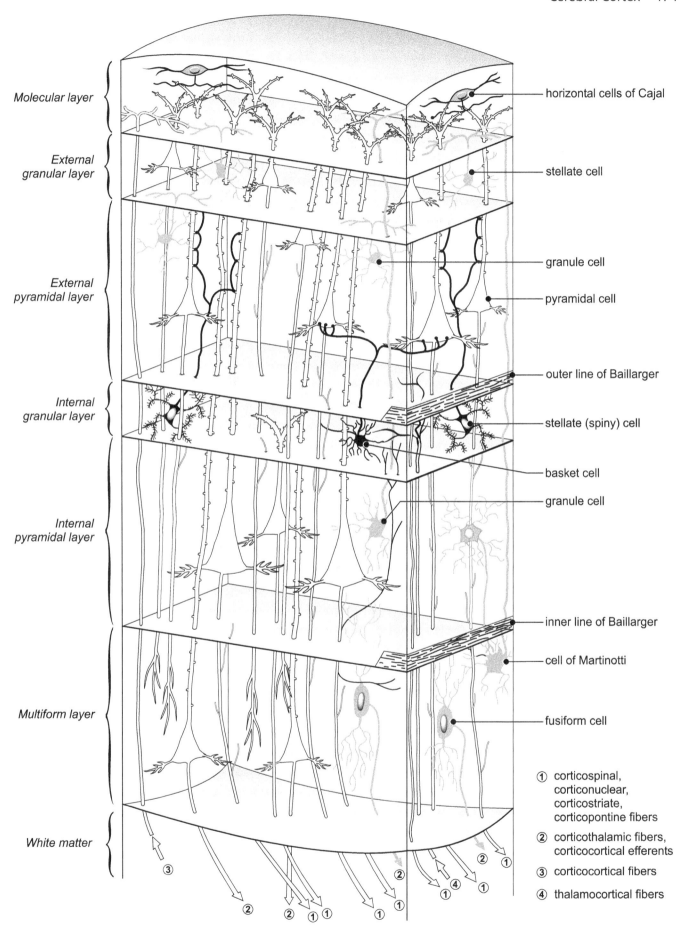

Figure 14.1   Histology of the cerebral cortex

iii. *stellate cells*, *basket cells* and *cells of Martinotti*
- are interneurons

b. *Cortical Layers*:

The following account is restricted to the major features of the layers (Figure 14.1). The six layers, starting at the surface, are as follows:

1. *Molecular layer*: INPUT layer
   - consists of dendrites and axons
   - is the synaptic field of the cortex

11. *External granular layer:* INPUT layer
   - consists of interneurons

111. *External pyramidal layer:* OUTPUT layer
   - consists of pyramidal neurons
   - axons of pyramidal neurons project as association and projection fibers

1V. *Internal granular layer:* INPUT layer
   - consists of interneurons

V. *Internal pyramidal layer:* OUTPUT layer
   - consists of large pyramidal neurons (Betz cells in motor cortex)

V1. *Multiform layer:* OUTPUT layer
   - consists of interneurons and output axons

3. Functional Localization:

Different parts of the cortex are specialized for specific functions. The various functional areas of the cerebral cortex are:

A. General Somatic Sensation:

1. **Primary Somesthetic Area:** in postcentral gyrus and paracentral lobule (posterior part)

Connections (Figure 14.2):

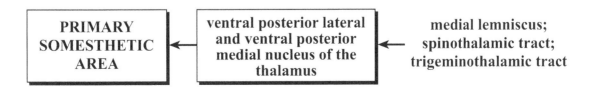

The map of the body, as indicated in Figure 7.1, is known as the ***homunculus.*** Various regions of the *contralateral* half of the body is represented as *inverted*. The body is represented disproportionately, determined by the functional importance of the area with reference to sensory function. The pharynx, tongue and jaw are represented in the most ventral portion of the primary somesthetic area, followed in ascending order by the face, hand, arm, trunk and thigh. The leg and foot are represented in the extension of the somesthetic area on the medial surface of the cerebral hemisphere.

function: discrimination of position and intensity of sensation of the opposite side of the body

Clinical Notes: Lesions of the primary somesthetic area results in: a) poor localization of stimulus b) vague awareness of pain and temperature.

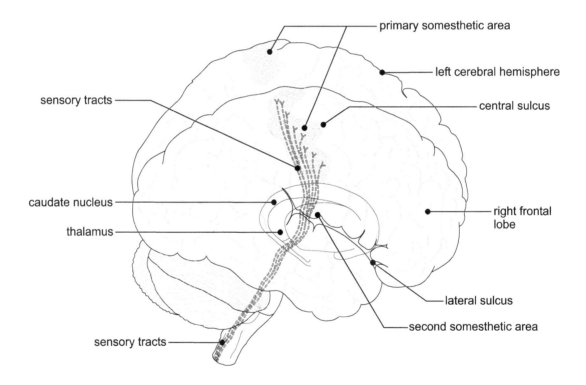

Figure 14.2   Primary sensory area of the cerebral cortex

2. ***Second Somesthetic Area:*** located in the dorsal wall of the lateral sulcus, in line with the postcentral gyrus

Connections:

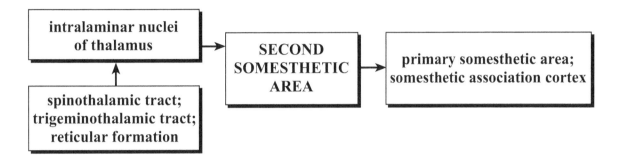

Various regions of the body are represented bilaterally, but contralateral projection predominates

function: involved in less discriminative aspects of sensation

3. ***Somesthetic Association Cortex:*** located in the precuneus and superior parietal lobule

Connections (Figure 14.3):

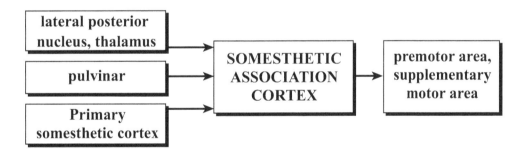

function: recognition, touch & identification

Clinical Notes: a lesion of the somesthetic association cortex results in:
- *astereognosis* or loss of spatial relationship of parts of the contralateral side of the body
- *tactile agnosia* or inability to identify objects with reference to shape and texture (in the absence of visual input)

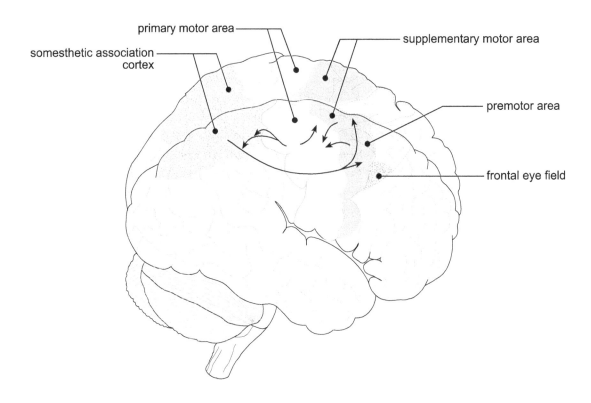

Figure 14.3   Functional areas of the cerebral cortex

4. ***Primary Visual Area***: occupies the calcarine sulcus and extends to the occipital pole

   Connections:

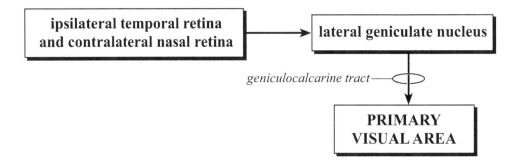

   function: left half of the visual field is represented in the right visual cortex and vice versa

   Clinical Notes: Lesions that affect the visual cortex of one hemisphere result in loss of vision in the contralateral half of the visual field

5. **Visual Association Area** - surrounds the calcarine sulcus; lateral and inferior surfaces of occipital lobe; posterior part of parietal lobe and lateral and inferior parts of temporal lobe. Also includes the inferior temporal gyrus and occipitotemporal gyri

Connections:

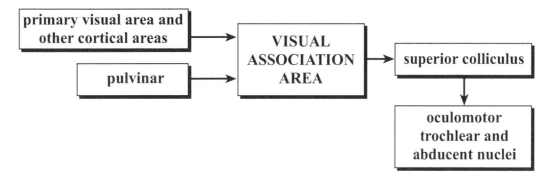

functions: relates present to past visual experiences; recognition and appreciation of what is seen

Visual information from visual association areas proceed anteriorly through two streams or paths. These are the **dorsal stream** and **ventral stream** (Figure 14.4).

   a. The **dorsal stream** (**"where" pathway**) extends from the superior part of occipital lobe and the posterior part of parietal lobe to the postcentral gyrus. The dorsal stream functions in analyzing movement and spatial relation of objects
   b. The **ventral stream** (**"what" pathway**) extends from the inferior parts of occipital and temporal lobes and functions in visual identification of objects and faces
   c. The inferior temporal gyrus and occipitotemporal gyri function in visual memories

Clinical Notes:
   i. Bilateral lesions in the superior part of the occipital lobe causes visual disorientation or inability to recognize extent of visual field and to perceive moving objects
   ii. Bilateral lesions of the inferior temporal gyrus and occipitotemporal gyri results in **prosopagnosia** (inability to recognize familiar faces)

6. **Primary Auditory Area**: is located in Heschl's convolutions (transverse temporal gyri) of the superior temporal gyrus

Connections:

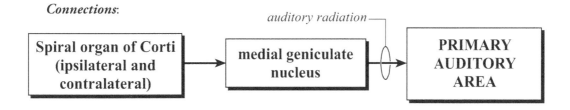

function: interprets pitch and rhythm of acoustic stimuli. Anterolateral part of the primary auditory area functions in low pitch and posteromedial part of the primary auditory area functions in high pitch

Clinical Notes:

   Bilateral lesion of the auditory association area results in impairment in interpreting complex combination of sounds

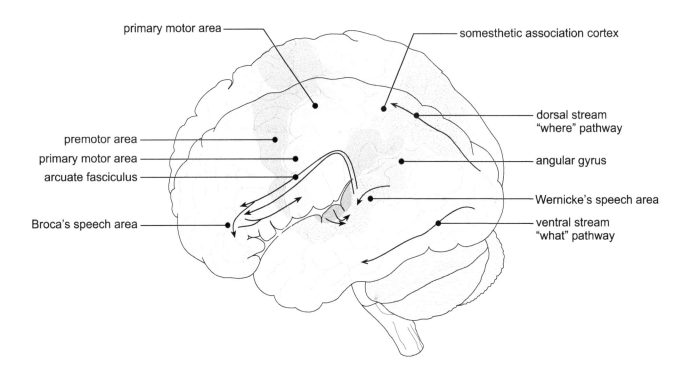

Figure 14.4   Motor and speech areas of the cerebral cortex

7. **Auditory association area:** is located in the planum temporale and posterior part of superior temporal gyrus. This is the Wernicke's area in the left hemisphere and is involved in *speech*

Connections:

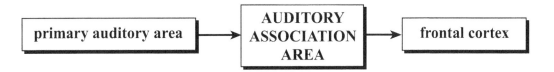

function: elaborate perception of acoustic information

8. **Taste** : located in the inferior part of the somesthetic area of the cortex and the insula

Connections:

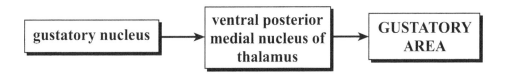

function: conscious awareness of gustatory stimuli

9. **Olfaction**: located in limen insulae, uncus and amygdaloid body

Connections:

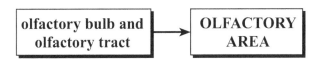

function: discrimination of different odors

10. **Vestibular *Cortex***: located at the posterior parietal lobe and insula

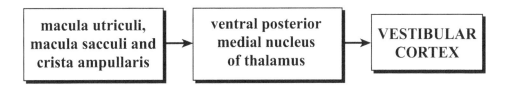

function: awareness of orientation of the body

B. Motor Cortex

1. ***Primary Motor Area:*** located in precentral gyrus and paracentral lobule (anterior part)

   Connections:

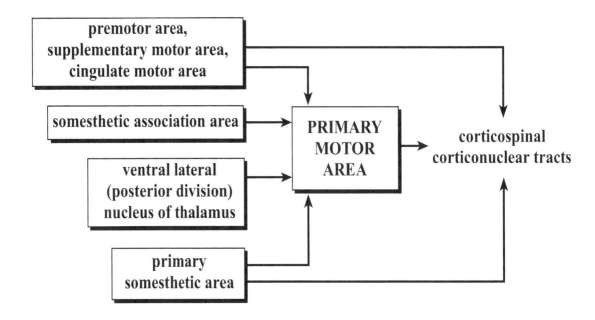

The map of the body as depicted in Figure 7.1 is known as the ***homunculus.*** Various regions of the contralateral half of the body is represented as inverted, similar to that of the primary somesthetic area (page 180)

function: execution of skilled movements

Clinical Notes:
Isolated lesions of the primary motor area results in weakness of the affected part of the contralateral side of the the body. Muscles are flaccid if the lesion is restricted to the precentral gyrus

2a. ***Supplementary Motor Area***: located on the medial surface of the frontal lobe, anterior to the paracentral lobule
  b. ***Cingulate Motor Area:*** located in the anterior half of the cingulate sulcus

Connections:

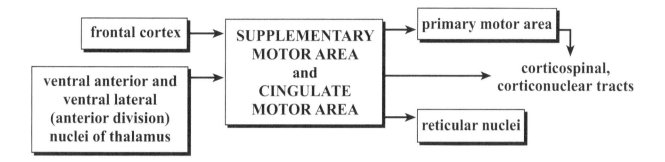

functions:

    a. the supplementary motor area is involved in retrieval of mental processes that precede motor tasks. The supplementary motor area is also necessary for normal speech

    b. the cingulate motor area is involved in anticipation of motor cognitive tasks

3. ***Premotor Area***: area of frontal lobe, anterior to the precentral gyrus

Connections:

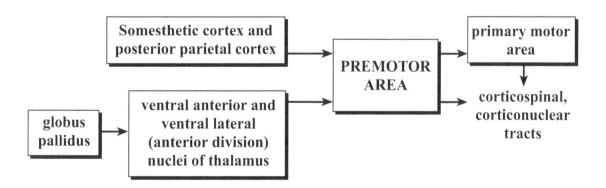

functions:

- directs the motor cortex
- involved in skilled motor activities of a complex and sequential nature

Clinical Notes:

    Lesions of the premotor area results in the inability to execute sequential and complex movements despite normal muscle function, referred to as ***apraxia.***

4. **Frontal Eye Field**: located in frontal lobe, anterior and inferior to the premotor area

Connections

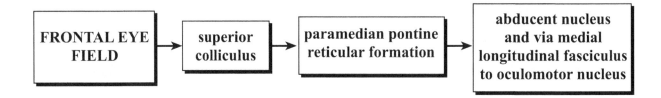

functions: involved in voluntary conjugate movements that cause deviation of eyes to the contralateral side

Clinical Notes:

Lesion of the frontal eye field causes the eye to deviate to the side of the lesion

5. **Prefrontal Cortex**: area of frontal lobe anterior to the premotor area

Connections:

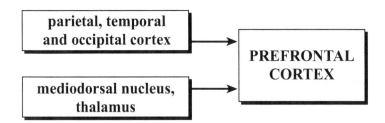

Functions: judgement, foresight and appropriate behavior

Clinical Notes:

Lesions of the prefrontal cortex leads to impairment in decision making and planning; alterations in social behavior are also observed

C. Language Areas: in the left hemisphere (Figure 14.4)

1. *Sensory Speech Area* or *Wernicke's Area*:

- located in the posterior part of the left superior temporal gyrus
- is the receptive language area and is important for understanding language
- it is connected to the visual association cortex for comphrension of words and with the angular gyrus for formation of words

2. *Broca's Area* or *Motor Speech Area*:
   * located in the left opercular & triangular areas of the inferior frontal gyrus
   * is important for production of speech
   * *arcuate fasciculus* connects the motor speech area and sensory speech area

Clinical Notes:

Lesions of language areas results in **aphasia** and involves many different disorders, only a few examples will be described

   i.   lesion of the sensory speech area results in *receptive aphasia* or failure to understand language, such as auditory and visual comphrension of language. Naming objects and formulating sentences are also affected
   ii. lesion of Broca's speech area results in *expressive aphasia* or distorted speech but comphrension of language is not affected
   iii. lesion of the supramarginal gyrus and arcuate fasciculus results in *conduction aphasia*. Speech is fluent with good comphrension of language but formulating and repetition of words are affected.
   iv. lesion of the occipital lobe and adjoining white matter results in *alexia* or the inability to read

CHAPTER
15

WHITE MATTER OF THE CEREBRUM

Overview

The inner white matter of the cerebrum consists of neuroglial cells and many afferent (corticopetal) and efferent (corticofugal) fibers. The largest source of afferents to the cerebral cortex are from the thalamus, including other regions, such as from the contralateral cerebral cortex, association cortex and from the brainstem. Efferent fibers are predominantly motor and project to various areas of the brain and spinal cord

1. Organization:

The white matter of the cerebrum can be classified as follows:

    a. ***Association fibers***: connect cortical areas of the ipsilateral cerebral hemisphere, conducting impulses between gyri of the ipsilateral hemisphere

    b. ***Commissural fibers***: connect similar cortical areas of the contralateral hemisphere, conducting impulses between similar functional areas of the hemispheres eg. corpus callosum

    c. ***Projection fibers:*** connect cortical areas with the diencephalon, brainstem or spinal cord. Projection fibers consist of ascending thalamocortical and descending cortical fibers

2. Pathways:

    a. ***Association Fibers***:

Prominent bundles of association fibers are indicated in Figure 15.1. These are:

        i. ***Cingulum:***
- courses within the cingulate gyrus
- interconnects cingulate gyrus, parahippocampal gyrus and septal area (limbic system)

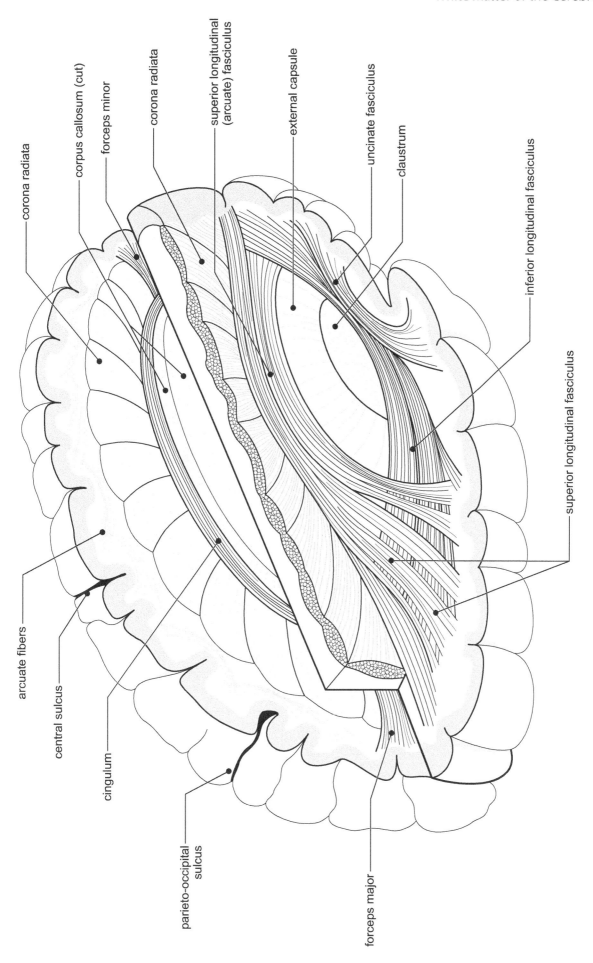

corona radiata

corpus callosum (cut)

forceps minor

corona radiata

superior longitudinal (arcuate) fasciculus

external capsule

uncinate fasciculus

claustrum

inferior longitudinal fasciculus

superior longitudinal fasciculus

arcuate fibers

central sulcus

cingulum

parieto-occipital sulcus

forceps major

Figure 15.1   Association fibers of the cerebrum

ii. *Superior longitudinal fasciculus* (*arcuate fasciculus)*
- connects cortices of the parietal, temporal and occipital lobes and the frontal lobe. For example, execution of specific movements involves sensory information from the parietal lobe to influence formulation of neuronal programs in the frontal lobe.
- also connects the sensory and motor language areas

iii. *Uncinate fasciculus:*
- connects the frontal and temporal lobes

b. **Commissural Fibers**:

i. *Corpus callosum:*
- largest fiber bundle in the human brain
- contains more than 300 million axons
- most of these fibers interconnect corresponding functional areas of both hemispheres
- the hand area of the primary somatosensory cortex and a large area of the primary visual area are not directly connected by commissural fibers
- the corpus callosum consists of the following parts, from anterior to posterior: *rostrum, genu, trunk* and *splenium* (Figure 15.2). The genu contains fibers that connect the frontal lobes, which comprise the *forceps minor* or *forceps frontalis* (Figure 15.1). The splenium contains fibers that connect the occipital lobes, which comprise the *forceps major* or *forceps occipitalis*.

  function: memory patterns exist for previous experiences and allows for interhemispheric transfer of learned tasks

Clinical Notes:
Commissurotomy affects transfer of information from one hemisphere to the other with respect to learned tasks and understanding language.

ii. *Anterior commissure*:
- crosses ventral to the corpus callosum and connects the temporal lobes of the cerebrum

iii. *Fornix*:
- connects the hippocampal formation (limbic system) to the mamillary body (hypothalamus) and septal area of the forebrain

- the fornix begins at the hippocampus as the *crura.* The crura curve forward and merge to form the *body* of the fornix and is located inferior to the trunk of the corpus callosum. The body of the fornix divides into *two* *columns* that extend ventrally and inferiorly to terminate in the mamillary bodies (Figure 17.1)

3. Projection Fibers:

A. *Internal capsule*:

Projection fibers are grouped together to form the *internal capsule*. The internal capsule fans out as the *corona radiata* in the white matter of the cerebrum (Figure 15.1). In horizontal sections, the internal capsule consists of three parts that are shaped as an arrowhead, directed towards the midline (Figure 12.2). The three parts of the internal capsule are the *anterior limb*, *genu* and *posterior limb.* In addition to the three parts, the *retrolenticular* and *sublenticular* portions of the internal capsule are located in relation to the lentiform nucleus.

Fibers in the internal capsule:

Comprise the *thalamic radiations* consisting of thalamocortical and corticothalamic circuits, including *cortical efferents* to the brainstem and spinal cord.

The following is a description of the location and type of fibers in the five portions of the internal capsule:

a. *anterior limb*: is located between the caudate nucleus and lentiform nucleus and contains the *anterior thalamic radiation*, which in turn contains:
   i. fibers from the mediodorsal nucleus $\Rightarrow$ prefrontal cortex
   ii. frontopontine fibers

b. *genu*: is located medial to the lentiform nucleus. The genu contains the *middle thalamic radiation*, which in turn contains:
   i. fibers from the ventral anterior, ventral lateral (anterior division) and ventral lateral (posterior division) of the thalamus $\Rightarrow$ premotor, primary motor cortex, supplementary motor area and cingulate motor area

c. *posterior limb*: is located between the lentiform nucleus and thalamus. It contains the *middle thalamic radiation*, which in turn contains:
   i. fibers from the ventral posterior lateral and ventral posterior medial nucleus of the thalamus $\Rightarrow$ primary sensory cortex
   ii. contains corticonuclear, corticospinal, frontopontine fibers

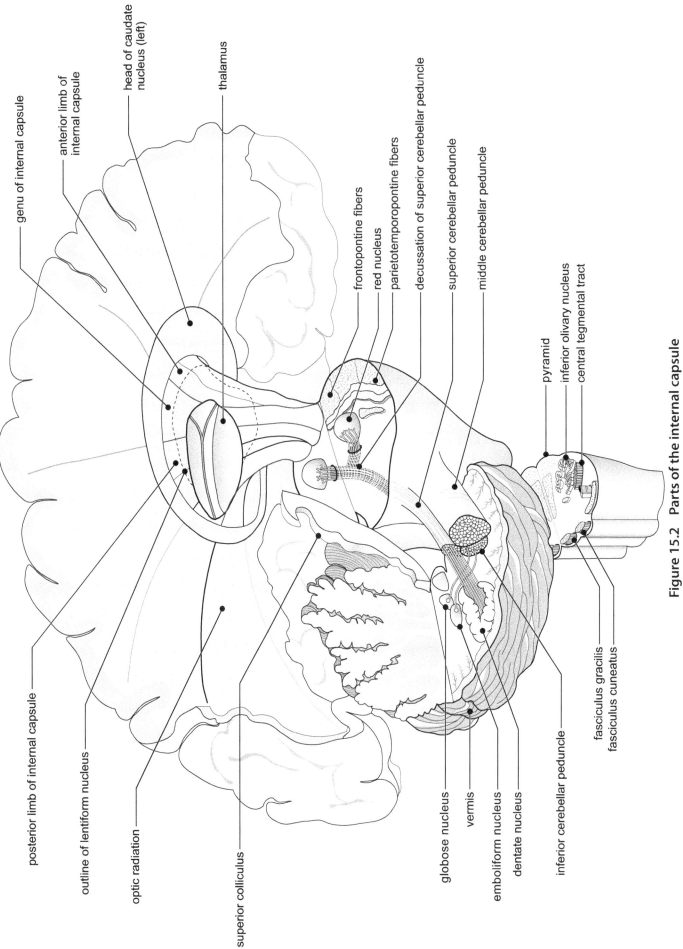

genu of internal capsule

anterior limb of internal capsule

head of caudate nucleus (left)

thalamus

frontopontine fibers

red nucleus

parietotemporopontine fibers

decussation of superior cerebellar peduncle

superior cerebellar peduncle

middle cerebellar peduncle

pyramid

inferior olivary nucleus

central tegmental tract

posterior limb of internal capsule

outline of lentiform nucleus

optic radiation

superior colliculus

globose nucleus

vermis

emboliform nucleus

dentate nucleus

inferior cerebellar peduncle

fasciculus gracilis

fasciculus cuneatus

Figure 15.2   Parts of the internal capsule

   d. *retrolentiform part*: is located behind the lentiform nucleus and contains
      the ***posterior thalamic radiation***, which in turn contains:
         i. geniculocalcarine tract

   e. *sublentiform part*: is located beneath the lentiform nucleus. It contains the
      inferior thalamic radiation which in turn contains:
         i. the auditory radiation, comprising fibers of the medial geniculate
             nucleus ⇒ primary auditory area of cerebral cortex

Clinical Notes:

A lesion in the posterior limb of the internal capsule results in an "***upper motor
neuron***" lesion. Symptoms are hemiplegia; spasticity and *Babinski sign*

CHAPTER
16

OLFACTORY SYSTEM

Overview

Olfactory sense is mediated by sensory neurons in the olfactory epithelium, located in the area of the superior nasal concha of the nasal cavity. Olfactory sensory cells project to neurons in the olfactory bulb, which in turn project via the olfactory tract to areas of the cortex. Olfactory sense is the only sense that relays directly to the cerebral cortex

I. Olfactory epithelium and nerves:

A. Olfactory epithelium consists of the following (Figure 16.1):

    i. olfactory neurosensory cells are **bipolar neurons** that function as sensory receptors. Each bipolar neuron consists of the following:
- **dendrite**, a short peripheral process that terminates into a bulbous **olfactory vesicle**, that is studded with long **cilia**. Cilia contain as many as 1,000 **odorant receptors** responsive to different odorant stimuli
- an unmyelinated **axon**, a longer process located at the opposite end of the bipolar neuron. Axons group together into bundles to form the **olfactory nerve**. Small bundles of olfactory nerves pass through the cribriform plate of the ethmoid to terminate in the **olfactory bulb**.

    ii. **supporting cells**:
- are interspersed between bipolar neurons
- provide support of the olfactory receptor cells and contribute secretions to the mucus layer overlying the epithelium

    iii. **basal cells:**
- divide to replace olfactory receptor cells that normally have a lifespan of one to two months.

    iv. **olfactory glands**:
- are located beneath the epithelium
- secretions renew the surface fluid and promote dissolution of odoriferous substances

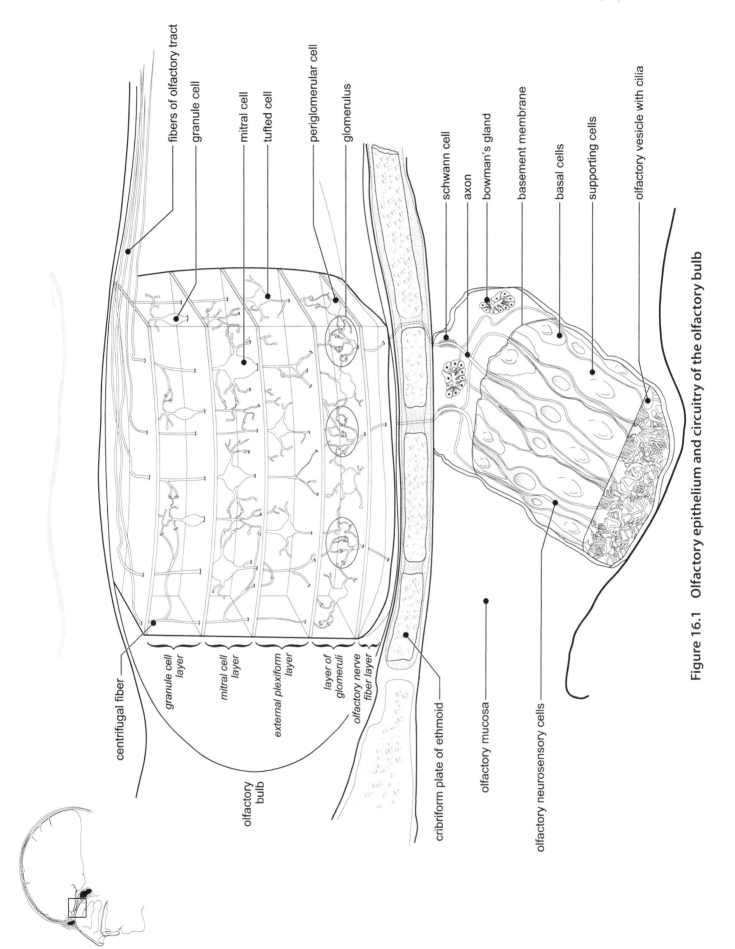

fibers of olfactory tract
granule cell
mitral cell
tufted cell
periglomerular cell
glomerulus
schwann cell
axon
bowman's gland
basement membrane
basal cells
supporting cells
olfactory vesicle with cilia

centrifugal fiber
olfactory bulb
granule cell layer
mitral cell layer
external plexiform layer
layer of glomeruli
olfactory nerve fiber layer
cribriform plate of ethmoid
olfactory mucosa
olfactory neurosensory cells

Figure 16.1   Olfactory epithelium and circuitry of the olfactory bulb

B. **Olfactory transduction**:

 i. reception: odorant molecules attach directly or are bound to a odorant-binding protein to receptor proteins on surface of cilia of olfactory neurons

 ii. transduction: cation channels open $\Rightarrow$ influx of Na^+ and Ca^{2+} ions $\Rightarrow$ depolarization of cell membrane and propagation of nerve impulse

II. Olfactory bulb

A. *Features*:

 i. is located ventral to the orbital surface of frontal lobe and is connected to the olfactory tract

 ii. contains 4 cell types arranged in five indistinct layers (Figure 16.1). The **mitral cells** and **tufted cells** are the principal cells of the olfactory bulb, **granule cells** and **periglomerular cells** are interneurons.

 iii. olfactory nerves enter the olfactory bulb to form synaptic configurations with dendrites of the mitral, tufted and periglomerular cells, termed *glomeruli* (Figure 16.1). The circuitry of the olfactory bulb is summarized in Fig.16.2.

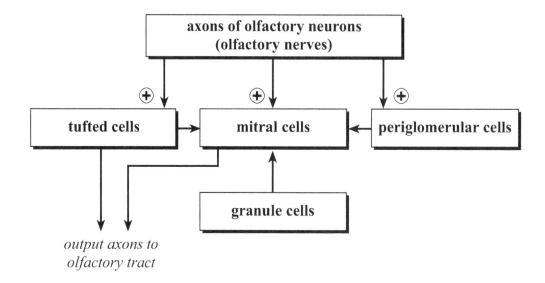

Figure 16.2   Circuitry of the olfactory bulb

B. *Circuitry of the Olfactory bulb* (Fig.16.2):

   i.   axons from all olfactory receptor neurons form excitatory axodendritic synapses on mitral, tufted and periglomerular cells. Tufted cells, periglomerular and granule cells also form dendrodendritic synapses with mitral cells. Mitral and tufted cells are excitatory neurons. The activity of the mitral and tufted cells are modified through lateral inhibitory synaptic connections of interneurons. This complex circuitry helps in identifying different odors.

   ii.   direct stimulation of receptors; convergence of many sensory receptors onto only one or two glomeruli in the ipsilateral olfactory bulb and specificity of neuronal circuits of the olfactory bulb account for low threshold and sensitivity to minute amounts of reactants in air.

III. Olfactory Tract:

   i.   is a narrow band, containing axons of mitral cells and tufted cells

   ii.   fibers of the olfactory tract separate at its caudal extremity, the **olfactory trigone**. Fibers separate into two bundles, the *lateral olfactory stria* and an *intermediate olfactory stria* (Fig.16.3).

IV. Olfactory Pathways:

   i.   Axons of mitral and tufted cells in olfactory bulb ⇒ olfactory tract ⇒ olfactory trigone ⇒ separate into lateral olfactory stria and intermediate olfactory stria (Figure 16.3)

   ii.   *lateral olfactory stria* disperse and terminate in the **lateral olfactory area** (*primary olfactory area*), which includes the *pyriform cortex* and the *amygdala* (Fig.16.4). The areas collectively termed the *pyriform cortex* comprise the *uncus*, *limen insulae* and the *entorhinal area* (anterior end of parahippocampal gyrus). The lateral olfactory area is responsible for conscious awareness of odors.

   iii.   *intermediate olfactory stria* terminate in the *anterior perforated substance*. The intermediate olfactory stria is poorly developed in humans.

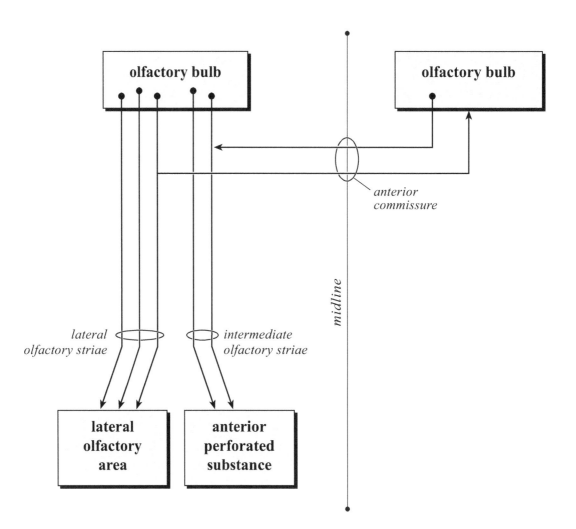

Figure 16.3   Schematic diagram of olfactory pathways

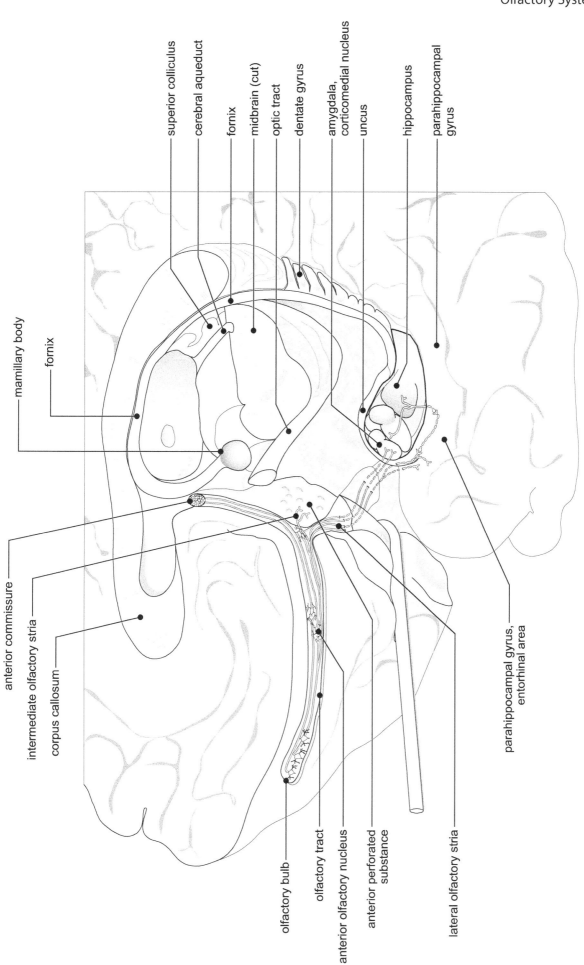

superior colliculus

cerebral aqueduct

fornix

midbrain (cut)

optic tract

dentate gyrus

amygdala, corticomedial nucleus

uncus

hippocampus

parahippocampal gyrus

mamillary body

fornix

anterior commissure

intermediate olfactory stria

corpus callosum

olfactory bulb

olfactory tract

anterior olfactory nucleus

anterior perforated substance

lateral olfactory stria

parahippocampal gyrus, entorhinal area

Figure 16.4   Central olfactory pathways

V. Central Pathways:

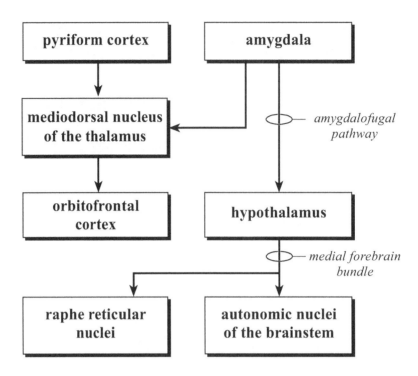

Figure 16.5   Schematic diagram of central pathways

In addition to the pathways directly related to the sense of smell, many projections to other cortical areas are necessary for somatic and visceral responses to smell. These connections are outlined in Fig.16.5

i. The primary olfactory area projects, via the mediodorsal nucleus of the thalamus to the ***orbitofrontal cortex*** (olfactory association cortex). The amygdala projects via the ***medial forebrain bundle*** to the hypothalamus. This connection plays a role in olfactory regulation of food intake.

ii. fibers of the medial forebrain bundle traverse the hypothalamus, project caudally and connect the hypothalamus to the autonomic nuclei of the brainstem and the raphe reticular nuclei. In addition, neurons of the entorhinal cortex project to the hippocampus via a fiber bundle, the ***perforant pathway*** (Figure 17.3). Through these pathways, specific aromas evoke autonomic responses, at times pleasurable, at other times not pleasurable.

VI. Clinical Notes:

a. upper respiratory infections or the common cold can cause temporary loss of olfactory function.

b. decrease in olfactory function occurs with normal aging. Decrease in olfactory sensitivity associated with *Alzheimer's* and *Parkinson's* diseases are associated with neuronal loss in the the amygdala

c. tumors located in the floor of the anterior cranial fossa, compressing the olfactory bulb or olfactory tract can cause loss of smell or ***anosmia***

d. lesions in the primary olfactory area, particularly the area around the uncus and the amygdala can cause ***uncinate fits***. Such olfactory hallucinations are characterized by imaginary disagreeable odor and involuntary movements of the lips and tongue

CHAPTER
17

LIMBIC SYSTEM

Overview

The limbic system consists of a network of structures that interconnect components of the cerebral hemispheres and the midbrain. The limbic system connects with the olfactory system, hypothalamus and cerebral cortex and are therefore involved in complex functions such as memory, instinct and emotions. The term *limbic system* emerged from the concept of the *limbic lobe*.

I. Limbic lobe:

- consists of a C-shaped ring of gray matter on the medial surface and basal parts of cerebral hemispheres
- three structures of the limbic lobe are the **septal area**, **cingulate gyrus** and *parahippocampal gyrus* (*subiculum*)

II. Limbic System:

- includes many structures
- comprises structures of the limbic lobe as well as cortical and subcortical structures connected to it
- plays a role in memory, visceral and motor responses

The structures of the limbic system include limbic lobe structures (*septal area*, *cingulate gyrus*, *parahippocampal gyrus*); *hippocampal formation*, *amygdaloid body*, *hypothalamus* and *lateral dorsal* and *anterior nuclei* of the *thalamus*.

The major components of the limbic system are the **hippocampal formation**, **amygdaloid complex** and the **septal area.** Each of these components are as follows:

A. HIPPOCAMPAL FORMATION:

1. *Features*:

- the hippocampal formation develops as a result of continuous expansion and infolding of the parahippocampal gyrus into the inferior horn of the lateral ventricle (Figure 17.1).

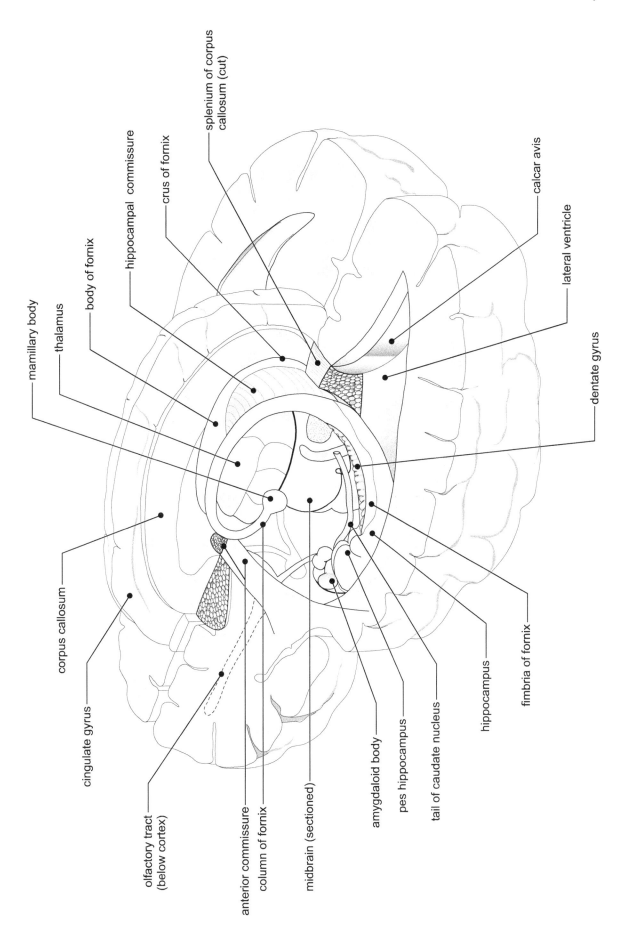

mamillary body

thalamus

body of fornix

hippocampal commissure

crus of fornix

splenium of corpus
callosum (cut)

calcar avis

lateral ventricle

dentate gyrus

corpus callosum

cingulate gyrus

olfactory tract
(below cortex)

anterior commissure

column of fornix

midbrain (sectioned)

amygdaloid body

pes hippocampus

tail of caudate nucleus

hippocampus

fimbria of fornix

Figure 17.1   Structures of the limbic system

- it is comprised of the **hippocampus**, **dentate gyrus** and *parahippocampal gyrus* (**subiculum**).
- it merges rostrally with the amygdaloid body and ventrally with the entorhinal cortex

2. **Anatomy:**

   i. *Hippocampus*: largest part of the hippocampal formation

   - is located on the floor of temporal horn of the lateral ventricle and covered by the parahippocampal gyrus
   - the anterior end is marked by digitations, referred to as *pes hippocampus*. In the sagittal plane, the hippocampus is cylindrical, extending to the caudal end of the corpus callosum (Figure 17.1).
   - appears C-shaped in coronal sections, resembling a ram's horn and hence referred to as *ammon's horn*
   - along the medial border of the hippocampus are afferents and efferents of the hippocampus that give rise to the *fimbria* of the hippocampus (Figure 17.1).
   - hippocampi are connected by commissural fibers (Figure 17.1)

   ii. *Dentate gyrus*:

   - its surface is toothed, hence the terminology
   - it is located between the hippocampus and the subiculum
   - in coronal sections, the hippocampus and the dentate gyrus appear as two interlocking C-shaped structures (Figure 17.2).

   iii. *Parahippocampal gyrus* (*subiculum*):

   - is a transition area between the hippocampus and the entorhinal cortex
   - it includes the posterior part of the parahippocampal gyrus
   - is important for flow of information into the hippocampus

3. **Cellular Organization of the hippocampal formation**:

   - the cortex of the three structures of the hippocampal formation, termed the *archicortex*, are arranged in three cell layers unlike that of the six-layered neocortex.
   - the hippocampus can be subdivided into three sectors or regions, termed *CA1*, *CA2*, *CA3* (Figure 17.2).
   - collaterals from axons of CA3 *pyramidal neurons,* referred to as *Schaffer collaterals,* project to CA1 sector. The pyramidal neurons in area CA1 are highly susceptible to oxygen deprivation. This region is referred to as *Sommer's sector.*

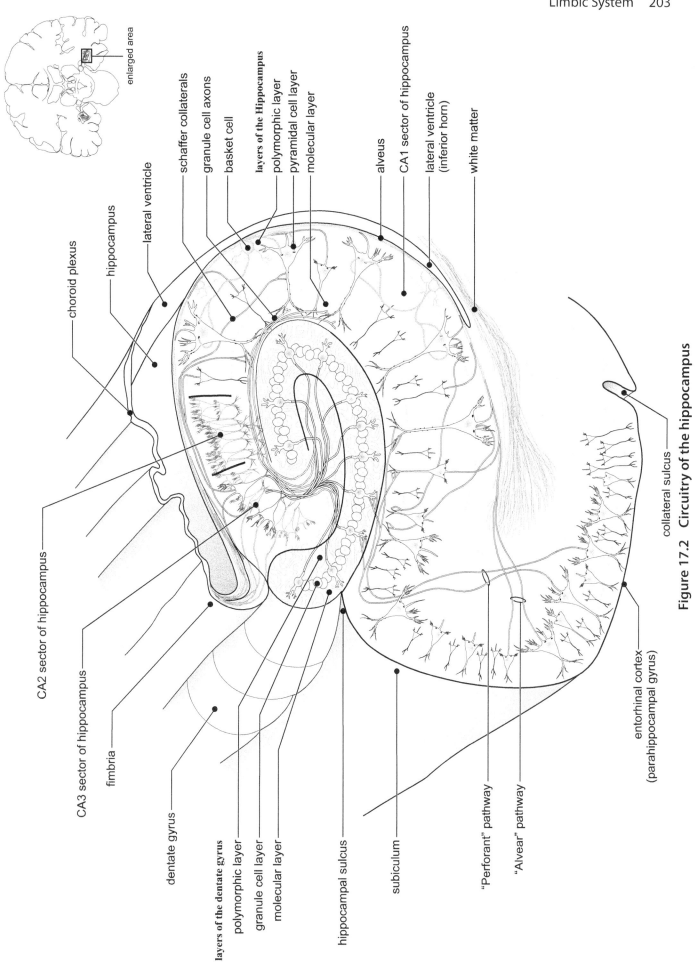

Figure 17.2   Circuitry of the hippocampus

enlarged area

choroid plexus

hippocampus

lateral ventricle

schaffer collaterals

granule cell axons

basket cell

layers of the Hippocampus
polymorphic layer
pyramidal cell layer
molecular layer

alveus

CA1 sector of hippocampus

lateral ventricle
(inferior horn)

white matter

collateral sulcus

CA2 sector of hippocampus

CA3 sector of hippocampus

fimbria

dentate gyrus

layers of the dentate gyrus
polymorphic layer
granule cell layer
molecular layer

hippocampal sulcus

subiculum

"Perforant" pathway

"Alvear" pathway

entorhinal cortex
(parahippocampal gyrus)

4. **Circuitry of the hippocampal formation**: consists of many afferent and efferent pathways

   A. **Afferent Pathways** (Figure 17.4):

   Major input is from the entorhinal cortex, reaching the hippocampal formation by two routes. These are:

      i. *Perforant path*:
      fibers from the entorhinal cortex, perforate the subiculum $\Rightarrow$ hippocampus and dentate gyrus (Figure 17.2)

      ii. *Alvear path*:
      fibers from entorhinal cortex $\Rightarrow$ enter through the white matter, forming the *alveus*, to terminate in the *CA1* sector of the hippocampus and in the subiculum (Figure 17.2)

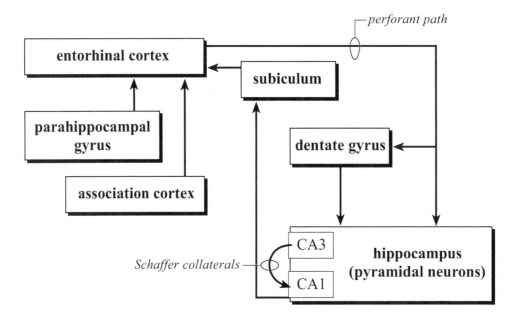

Figure 17.3   Schematic diagram of the afferent connections of the hippocampus

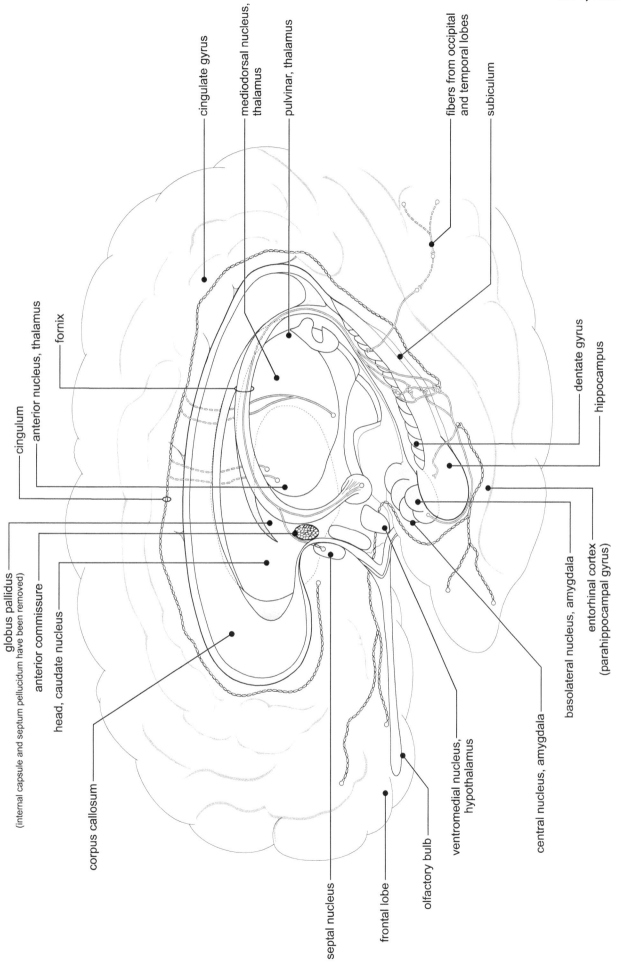

cingulate gyrus

mediodorsal nucleus, thalamus

pulvinar, thalamus

fibers from occipital and temporal lobes

subiculum

fornix

anterior nucleus, thalamus

cingulum

globus pallidus
(internal capsule and septum pellucidum have been removed)

anterior commissure

head, caudate nucleus

corpus callosum

septal nucleus

frontal lobe

olfactory bulb

ventromedial nucleus, hypothalamus

central nucleus, amygdala

basolateral nucleus, amygdala

entorhinal cortex (parahippocampal gyrus)

hippocampus

dentate gyrus

Figure 17.4 Afferents of the hippocampus

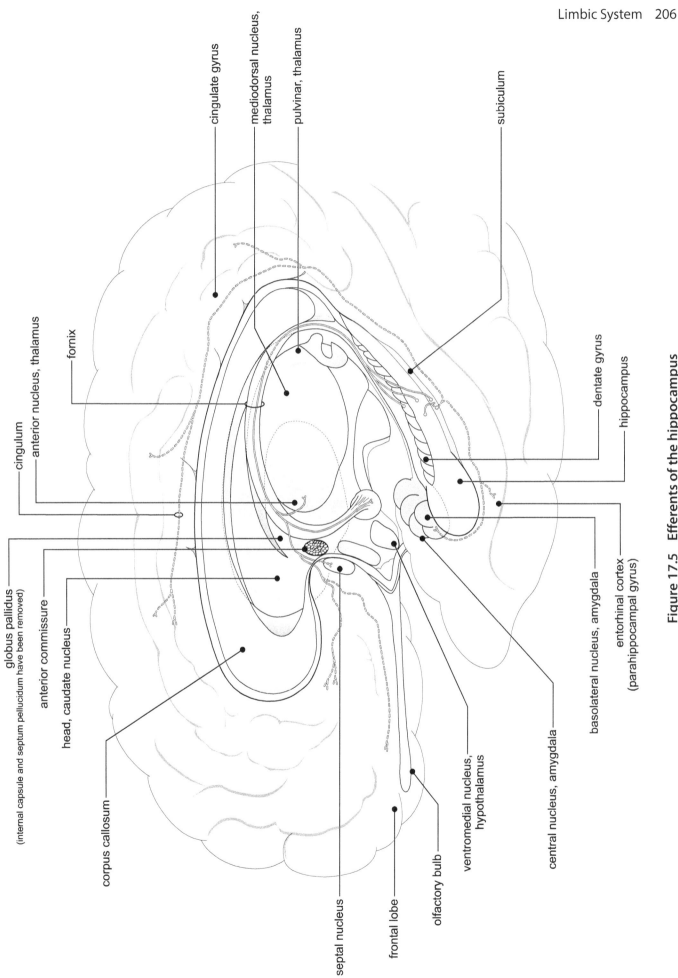

cingulate gyrus

mediodorsal nucleus, thalamus

pulvinar, thalamus

subiculum

fornix

anterior nucleus, thalamus

cingulum

dentate gyrus

hippocampus

globus pallidus
(internal capsule and septum pellucidum have been removed)

anterior commissure

head, caudate nucleus

basolateral nucleus, amygdala

entorhinal cortex
(parahippocampal gyrus)

corpus callosum

ventromedial nucleus, hypothalamus

central nucleus, amygdala

septal nucleus

frontal lobe

olfactory bulb

Figure 17.5   Efferents of the hippocampus

The entorhinal-hippocampal circuitry is a closed loop of connections that involves a four synapse pathway (Figure 17.3). Information that originates and terminates with the entorhinal cortex is as follows:

    a. from entorhinal cortex (via perforant path) ⇒ dentate gyrus and hippocampus

    b. neurons in dentate gyrus synapse with ⇒ CA3 pyramidal neurons

    c. axons (*Schaffer collaterals*) of CA3 pyramidal neurons synapse with ⇒ CA1 pyramidal neurons

    d. CA1 pyramidal neurons ⇒ synapse in subiculum ⇒ to project back to entorhinal cortex

iii. afferent fibers travel in the **fornix** and relay from the:

- contralateral hippocampus and septal area
- thalamic nuclei
- hypothalamic nuclei

B. *Efferent Pathways*:

  i. from hippocampus ⇒ subiculum

  ii. hippocampus; subiculum ⇒ entorhinal cortex ⇒ sensory areas and sensory association cortex

  iii. *Fornix:* is the largest output tract (Figures 17.5 and 17.6). The pathway is as follows:

    a. arise from pyramidal neurons of the hippocampus, originating at the ventricular surface of the hippocampus as the *alveus*.

    b. alveus forms a flattened band, the *fimbria*.

    c. fimbria continue posteriorly, arching beneath the splenium of the corpus callosum to form the *crus of the fornix.*

    d. the two crura merge in the midline to form the *body of the fornix*

    e. each body of the fornix is linked by a thin band of fibers, the *commissure of the hippocampus* (Figure 17.1)

f. body of the fornix extends to the *interventricular foramen,* where it separates into the **columns of the fornix.**

g. columns of the fornix arch inferiorly, separating at the anterior commissure into **precommissural** and **postcommissural fibers.**

h**. precommissural fibers** terminate in the **septal nuclei** and **hypothalamus** (anterior part)

i. **postcommissural fibers,** the bulk of the fornix, descend through the hypothalamus and terminate in the **mamillary bodies** and the **lateral dorsal nucleus** of the thalamus

iv. **Functional Significance**:

The entorhinal cortex receives many projections, directly from the olfactory cortex and indirectly from many sensory association areas of the cortex. The entorhinal cortex in turn conveys information from the cortex to the hippocampus. Thus the entorhinal area serves as an important connection between the cerebral cortex and hippocampus and the many connections play an important role in allowing a particular smell to evoke memories of a particular place or event.

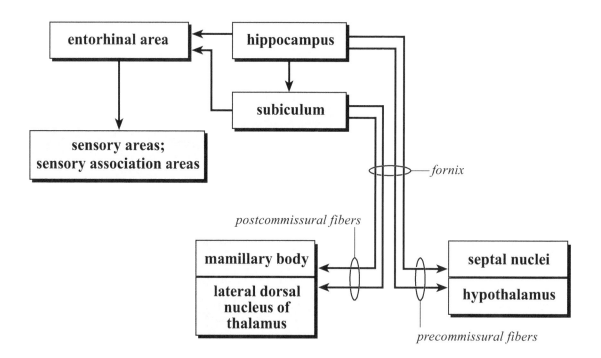

Figure 17.6   Schematic diagram of efferent connections of the hippocampus

5. **Limbic System and its connections**:

A. *Circuit of Papez*:

1. is a ring of tracts interconnecting structures of the limbic system, originating and terminating in the hippocampus. It connects limbic structures with the neocortex and the hypothalamus.

2. sequence of components of the ***Circuit of Papez*** are indicated in Figure 17.7 and include the following:

a. information flows from the hippocampus via the fornix to the mamillary body. The mamillary body project, via the *mamillothalamic tract*, to the anterior nucleus of thalamus, which in turn connect to the cingulate gyrus.

b. information from the cingulate gyrus project, via the *cingulum*, to the entorhinal cortex, which in turn projects back to the hippocampus.

Functional significance:

The Circuit of Papez connects limbic structures with the hypothalamus and the neocortex. Output from the hippocampus, via the fornix, to the hypothalamus elicits endocrine and autonomic responses. Connection of the limbic system with the cerebral cortex plays a role in controlling emotional behaviors.

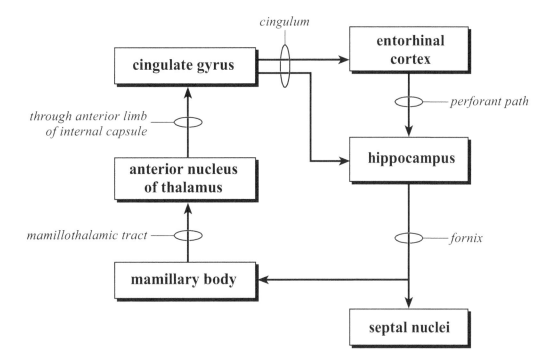

Figure 17.7   Schematic diagram of the Circuit of Papez

6. **Functions of the hippocampal formation**:

Memory:

- hippocampal circuits are involved in consolidating **short term** (or immediate) memory into **long term memory**.
- newly learned information is stored in short-term memory, and if reinforced, stored into long-term memory.
- long-term memory (Figure. 17.8) includes **explicit** (or **declarative**) **memory** and **implicit** (or **procedural**) **memory**.
- explicit memory can be consciously recalled while procedural memory includes memories of procedures and skills
- the process of ***long-term potentiation*** or formation of neuronal synaptic contacts is the mechanism by which short-term memory is assembled into long-term memory.

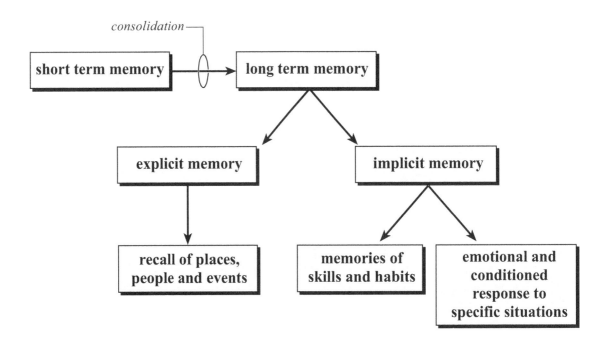

Figure 17.8 Types of memory

B. AMYGDALOID BODY (AMYGDALA):

1. Anatomy:

- is a major component of the limbic system
- almond-shaped, located at the rostral end of the hippocampus and anterior to the tail of caudate nucleus
- is at the tip of the temporal lobe, deep to the cortex of the uncus (Figure 17.9)
- consists of three principal nuclear groups

2. *Pathways*:

A. *Afferents* to the amygdaloid complex (figure 17 .9) are from:

    i. olfactory cortex, temporal lobe, frontal lobe,
    ii. hypothalamus
    iii. thalamus

functional significance: receives somatosensory, auditory, visual information from multimodal association areas of the cortex

B. *Efferents* from the amygdaloid complex (figure 17.10) are:

    i) *stria terminalis*:

- it arises from the amygdaloid complex
- courses dorsally and ventrally along the curve of the tail of the caudate nucleus
- terminates in the septal nuclei and anterior hypothalamus
- fibers from the stria terminalis travel via the medial forebrain bundle to the nuclei of the brainstem

    ii) *ventral amygdalofugal pathway*:

- originates from the nuclear groups of the amygdaloid complex (figure 17.11)
- terminates in prefrontal cortex, mediodorsal nucleus of thalamus, hypothalamus, autonomic nuclei of brainstem

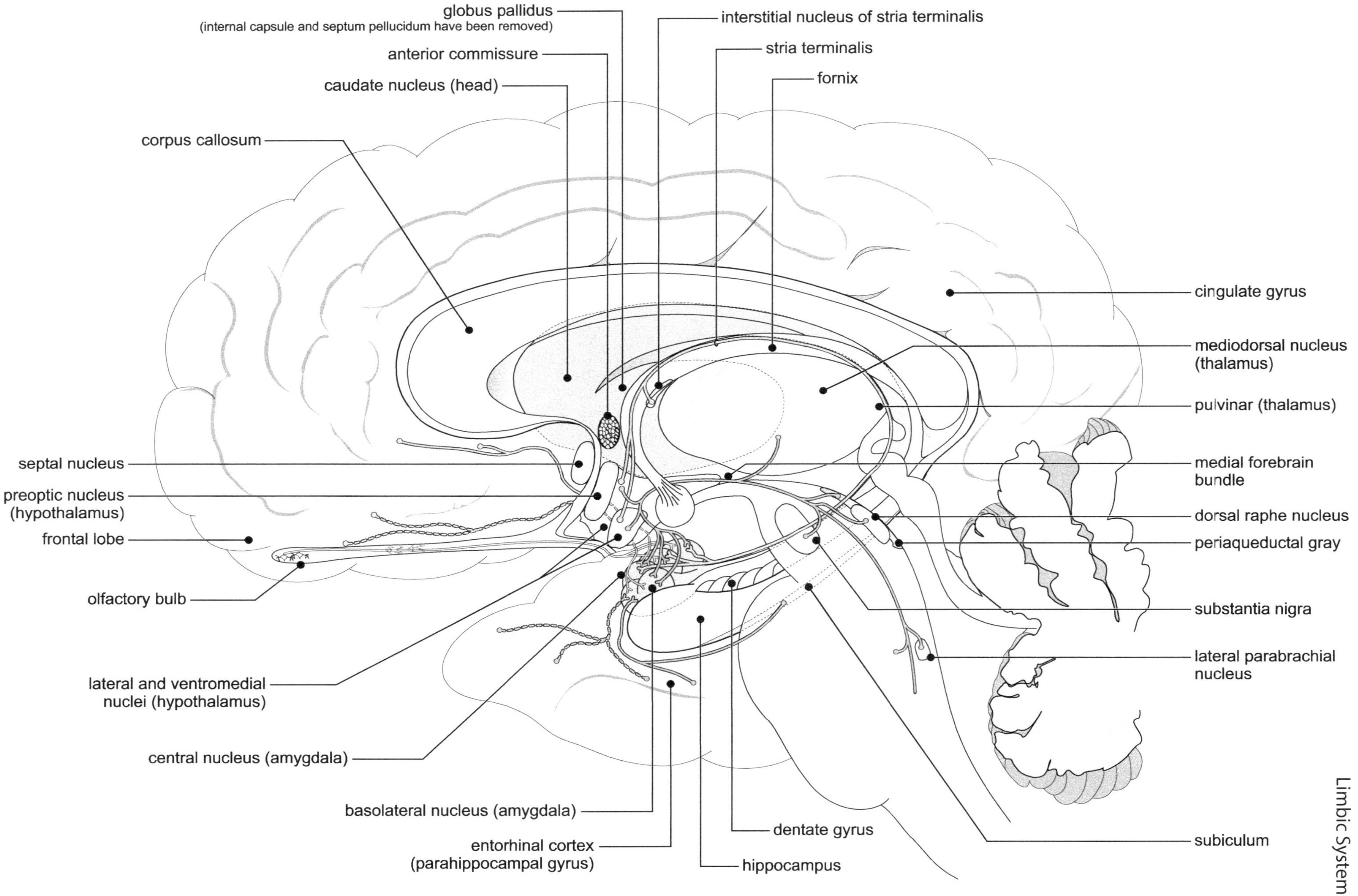

cingulate gyrus

mediodorsal nucleus (thalamus)

pulvinar (thalamus)

medial forebrain bundle

dorsal raphe nucleus

periaqueductal gray

substantia nigra

lateral parabrachial nucleus

subiculum

interstitial nucleus of stria terminalis

stria terminalis

fornix

dentate gyrus

hippocampus

globus pallidus
(internal capsule and septum pellucidum have been removed)

anterior commissure

caudate nucleus (head)

basolateral nucleus (amygdala)

entorhinal cortex (parahippocampal gyrus)

lateral nucleus (amygdala)

corpus callosum

lateral and ventromedial nuclei (hypothalamus)

central nucleus (amygdala)

septal nucleus

preoptic nucleus (hypothalamus)

frontal lobe

olfactory bulb

Figure 17.9   Afferents of the amygdala

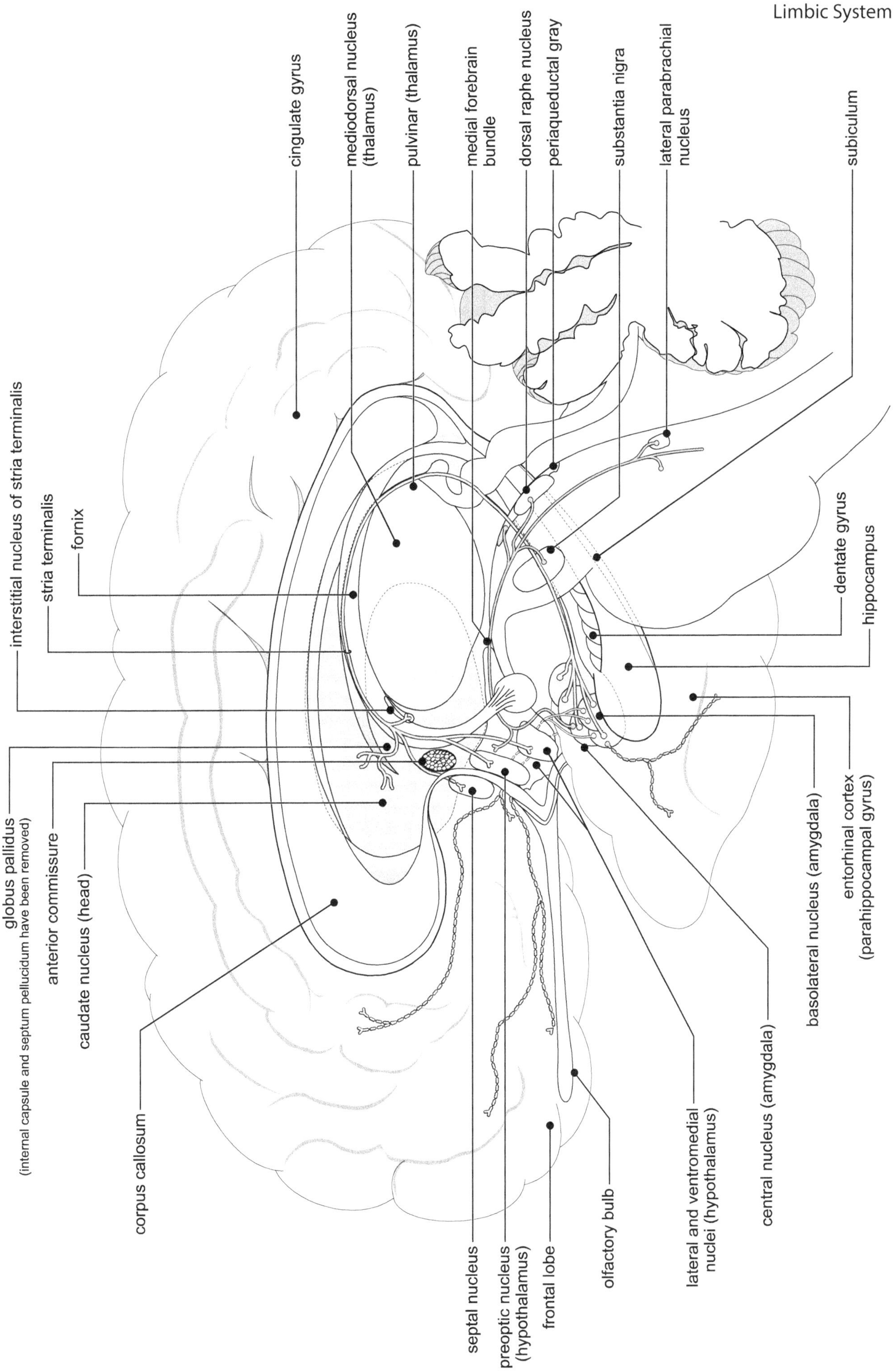

cingulate gyrus

mediodorsal nucleus (thalamus)

pulvinar (thalamus)

medial forebrain bundle

dorsal raphe nucleus

periaqueductal gray

substantia nigra

lateral parabrachial nucleus

subiculum

interstitial nucleus of stria terminalis

stria terminalis

fornix

dentate gyrus

hippocampus

globus pallidus
(internal capsule and septum pellucidum have been removed)

anterior commissure

caudate nucleus (head)

entorhinal cortex (parahippocampal gyrus)

basolateral nucleus (amygdala)

corpus callosum

central nucleus (amygdala)

lateral and ventromedial nuclei (hypothalamus)

septal nucleus

preoptic nucleus (hypothalamus)

frontal lobe

olfactory bulb

Figure 17.10   Efferents of the amygdala

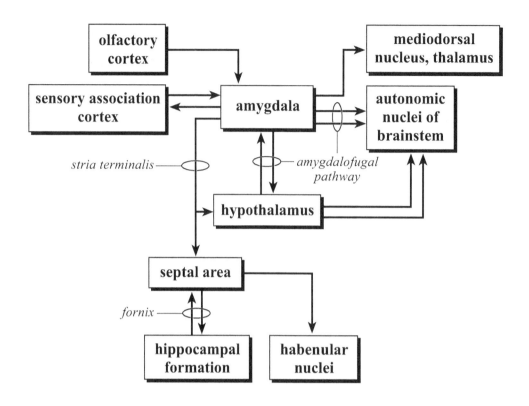

Figure 17.11   Schematic diagram of the connections of the amygdala

3. **Functions of the Amygdala**:

- amygdala integrates sensory information received from association areas of the cortex to link a particular stimuli to a particular emotion, such as, object recognition with fear eg. coming face-to-face with a bear
- by connecting diverse sensory areas of the cortex with the hypothalamus and brainstem autonomic centers, the amygdala helps to integrate autonomic responses (behavioral expression) that occur with particular emotions such as anger or fear
- also involved in motivation and behaviors essential to survival, such as feeding and reproduction

C. SEPTAL AREA:

1. **Anatomy**:

- consists of *septal nuclei*
- located on the medial surface of the hemisphere, rostral to the anterior commissure (Figure 17-10)

2. **Pathways**:

    a. *Afferents and Efferents* are:

        The septal area has reciprocal connections with the following areas:
           i. hippocampus, via the ***fornix***
           ii. amygdala, via the ***stria terminalis***
           iii. hypothalamus and brainstem tegmentum, via the ***medial forebrain bundle***
           iv. habenular nuclei via the ***stria medullaris thalami***

    b**. Functional Significance**:

- regulates activity of the hippocampus
- evokes behaviors in response to environmental stimuli

III. Clinical correlations with damage to components of the limbic system:

    i. *amnesia*: bilateral lesion of the hippocampus causes anterograde amnesia or inability to retain or learn new information. The *Sommer's sector* is sensitive to oxygen deprivation and is the first to be affected with decrease blood supply to the hippocampus

    ii. *temporal lobe epilepsy*: caused by propagation of abnormal action potentials through limbic connections, which are characterized by subjective visceral sensations (or aura) leading to convulsions or loss of consciousness.

    iii. *korsakoff's syndrome*: loss of memory of recent events brought about by prolonged thiamine deficiency caused by chronic alcoholism

    iv. *Kluver-Bucy syndrome*: experiments performed in animals have shown that bilateral lesions of the medial part of the temporal lobe involving the amygdala causes docility and hypersexuality

CHAPTER
18

VISUAL SYSTEM

Overview

Vision is the most important sense in the human. The visual system is important for recognition and location of objects, control of eye movements and postural control with reference to movement. The visual system consists of the eyeball, optic nerve and the pathways from the retina to the cortex.

The following description of the visual system is restricted to the major features of the eye and the visual pathways to the cortex.

I. Anatomy of the Eyeball

A. The eyeball is located within the orbital cavity and consists of the following parts when viewed anteriorly (Figure 18.1):

    i. *cornea*
- is an outer, transparent disc that covers the iris
- focuses light

    ii. *iris*
- is a pigmented layer with a central opening, the pupil

B. A horizontal section of the eyeball shows the following parts (Figure 18.1):

    i. *sclera:*
- outer fibrous covering that forms the "white" of the eye
- provides support and shape
- is pierced posteriorly by the optic nerve

    ii. *choroid:*
- middle, vascular layer

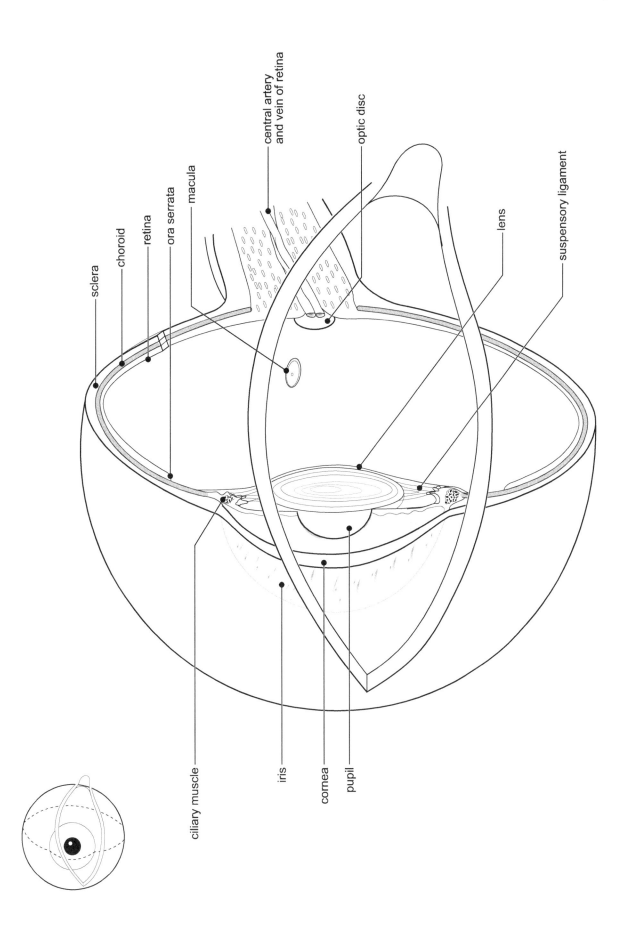

Figure 18.1   Structure of the eye

    iii. *retina:*
- innermost light sensitive layer
- develops as an outgrowth of the diencephalon, the **optic vesicle** and is connected to it by the **optic stalk**
- the optic vesicle invaginates to form a two-layered **optic cup**
- the optic cup gives rise to the *retina.* The outer of the two layers is the **pigment epithelium** and the inner layer is the **neural layer**. The optic stalk becomes the *optic nerve*
- the retina terminates anteriorly as the **ora serrata**
- the **optic disk** (blind spot) is the region of exit of the optic nerve
- the **macula lutea** is the central area of the retina and does not contain large blood vessels
- the **fovea** is a depression in the center of the macula, an area for acuity of vision
- the **foveola**, located in the center of fovea, contains only cone receptors

C. *Layers of the Retina*

Consists of the following:

    i. *Pigment epithelium*:
- is the outer layer, adjacent to the choroid
- it consists of a single layer of pigmented cells
- it plays a role in decreasing scattering of light

    ii. *Neural layer*:
- consists of photoreceptors, the **rods** and **cones** (Figure 18.2)
- also contains bipolar cells, ganglion cells, association neurons and neuroglial cells

Clinical Note:
Detachment of the Retina: The two layers of the retina are not firmly connected. Trauma, such as a blow to the eye, can result in separation of the two layers as a result of fluid build-up between the two layers. Detachment of the retina, if untreated can lead to blindness.

D. **Neural layer of the Retina**:

    1. *Neurons and layers* (Figure 18.2):

The neural layer of the retina is arranged in six layers and the arrangement of the various components, from superficial to deep, are as follows:

    i. **rods** and **cones** with specialized glial cells (**Muller cells**) interspersed between the photoreceptors

ii. a narrow *synaptic zone*, in which photoreceptors synapse with ***bipolar neurons*** and with laterally spreading processes of ***horizontal cells*** and ***interplexiform cells***

iii. a layer of ***amacrine cells***

iv. a *synaptic zone*, in which bipolar cells synapse with ***ganglion cells*** and laterally spreading processes of ***amacrine cells*** and ***interplexiform cells***

v. a layer of ***ganglion cells***

vi. axons of ganglion cells group together to form the ***optic nerve***

2. ***Photoreceptors:***

   a. ***Rods***:
      - 130 million
      - increases peripherally
      - absent in foveola (center of fovea)

      functions in dim light and important for peripheral vision

   b. ***Cones:***
      - 7 million
      - decreases peripherally
      - increases in fovea (100,000)

      functions in visual detail and color vision

   c. ***Structure of rods and cones***:

      i. ***outer segment***:
         - is a double layered membranous discs
         - rods contain rhodopsin, which comprises of opsin and retinal (derivative of vitamin A)
         - cones (3 types) contain cone pigment that absorb either red, green or blue light

      ii. ***inner segment***:
         - is thicker in cone
         - contain organelles; neurofibrils and vesicles

      iii. ***rod fiber or cone fiber***
         - cone fiber is thicker than rod fiber and synapses with bipolar and association neurons

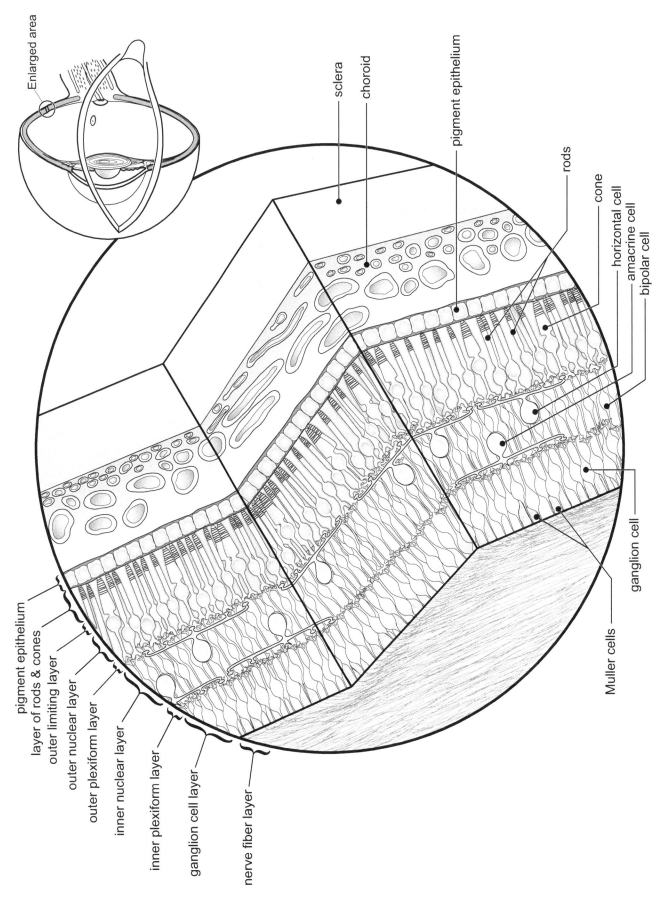

Enlarged area

sclera

choroid

pigment epithelium

rods

cone

horizontal cell

amacrine cell

bipolar cell

pigment epithelium

ganglion cell

Muller cells

pigment epithelium

layer of rods & cones

outer limiting layer

outer nuclear layer

outer plexiform layer

inner nuclear layer

inner plexiform layer

ganglion cell layer

nerve fiber layer

Figure 18.2   Structure of the retina

3. Pathway of stimulus

Stimulus (light) passes through the cornea, lens and the chambers of the eye to reach the photoreceptors in the retina. Figure 18.3 indicates the connections between cells of the retina. Lateral inhibition provided by interneurons enhance central transmission and enhances contrast between dark and illuminated regions of the retina.

i. *In darkness*:
   - Na⁺ channels are open and the photoreceptors are always partially depolarized
   - there is continuous release of inhibitory neurotransmitter onto bipolar cells

ii. *In light:*
   - Na⁺ channels close producing a hyperpolarized receptor potential
   - release of inhibitory neurotransmitter ceases
   - photoreceptors form excitatory synapses onto bipolar cells
   - bipolar cells, in turn, contact ganglion cells

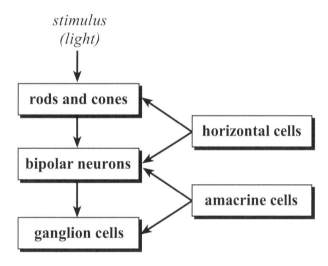

Figure 18.3   Schematic diagram of the connections of the cells of the retina

II. Visual field projection:

i. left visual field projects to the right lateral geniculate nucleus and to the right visual cortex
ii. right visual field projects to the left lateral geniculate nucleus and to the left visual cortex

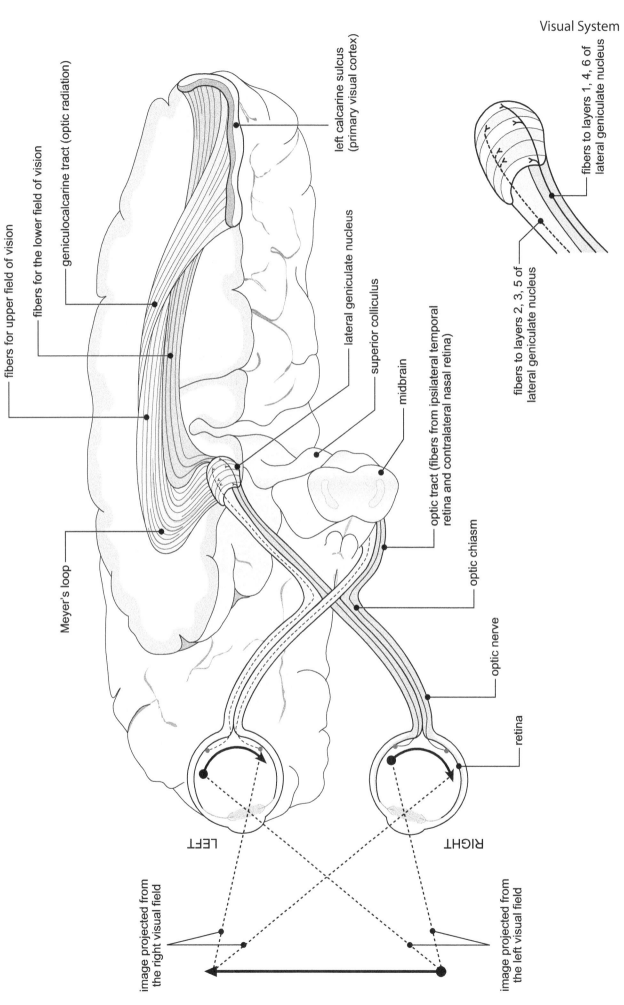

left calcarine sulcus
(primary visual cortex)

geniculocalcarine tract (optic radiation)

fibers for the lower field of vision

fibers for upper field of vision

lateral geniculate nucleus

superior colliculus

midbrain

optic tract (fibers from ipsilateral temporal
retina and contralateral nasal retina)

optic chiasm

optic nerve

retina

Meyer's loop

fibers to layers 1, 4, 6 of
lateral geniculate nucleus

fibers to layers 2, 3, 5 of
lateral geniculate nucleus

LEFT

RIGHT

image projected from
the right visual field

image projected from
the left visual field

Figure 18.4 Visual pathway from the retina to the calcarine sulcus

III. Projection from retina - *image is inverted and reversed*

a. lower 1/2 of   ⇒   upper   ⇒   medial part,
   visual field   half   lateral geniculate nucleus
                           of
                           retina   ⇓

                                       anterior 2/3 of visual cortex
                                       above calcarine sulcus

b. upper 1/2 of   ⇒   lower   ⇒   lateral part,
   visual field   half   lateral geniculate nucleus
                           of
                           retina   ⇓

                                       anterior 2/3 of visual cortex
                                       below calcarine sulcus

c. macula   ⇒   posterior region of lateral geniculate nucleus
                                            ⇓
                        posterior 1/3 of visual cortex (occipital pole)

IV. Visual Pathway (Figure 18.4)

From the retina (**ipsilateral temporal retina and contralateral nasal retina**) to:

optic nerve   ⇒   optic chiasm (fibers from the nasal half of the retina cross to the contralateral optic tract, fibers from the temporal 1/2 of retina pass through the ipsilateral optic tract)   ⇒   optic tract   ⇒   lateral geniculate nucleus   ⇒   geniculocalcarine tract   ⇒   traverses internal capsule, fibers of the upper half of the contralateral visual field loop into the temporal lobe as the ***Meyer's loop***   ⇒   primary visual cortex

V. Visual Reflexes

Pathways for accommodation and papillary light reflex have been described in Chapter 8. To summarize:

a. Pupillary light reflex
   retina ⇒ optic tract ⇒ olivary pretectal nucleus ⇒ *Edinger-Westphal nucleus* ⇒ oculomotor nerve

b. Accommodation reflex
   visual association area ⇒ superior colliculus ⇒ *Edinger-Westphal nucleus* ⇒ oculomotor nerve

Field of Left Eye   **Field of Right Eye**

① **lesion:** right optic nerve
defect: blindness in right eye

② **lesion:** optic chiasm, midline
defect: bitemporal hemianopia

③ **lesion:** right edge of optic chiasm
defect: right nasal hemianopia

④ **lesion:** right optic tract
defect: left homonymous hemianopia

⑤ **lesion:** right Meyer's loop
defect: left upper quadrant visual defect

⑥ **lesion:** right geniculocalcarine tract
defect: left homonymous hemianopia with sparing
of macular vision

LEFT

RIGHT

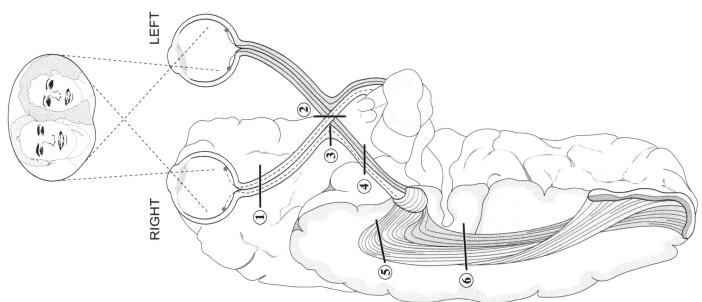

Figure 18.5 Visual field defects

c. Movement of head for fixation of gaze

visual association cortex $\Rightarrow$ superior colliculus $\Rightarrow$ cervical segments of spinal cord

VI. Visual Field defects

Refer to Figure 18.5 with reference to specific areas of lesions and functional deficits with respect to each lesion.

CHAPTER

19

AUDITORY AND VESTIBULAR SYSTEMS

AUDITORY SYSTEM

Overview

Hearing is one of the most important sensations. The auditory system is important in recognition and awareness of sounds, position of the head with reference to auditory stimuli and also for effective communication.

I. Anatomy of the Ear

The ear is composed of three parts, the external ear, the middle ear and the internal ear (Figure 19.1)

A. **External Ear:** directs sound waves towards the middle ear

Consists of the:
- *auricle*, the outer flap attached to the skull
- *external auditory meatus*, a curved tube that leads from the auricle to the tympanic membrane
- *tympanic membrane*, separates the external ear from the middle ear (Figure 19.1)

B. **Middle Ear:** an air-filled cavity in the temporal bone that consists of three ossicles and two small muscles that protect against excessive noise. The three ossicles (Figure 19.1) are the:
- **malleus**: is attached to the tympanic membrane and articulates with the incus
- **incus**: articulates with the stapes
- **stapes**: the foot plate of the stapes occupies the fenestra vestibuli (located between the middle ear and internal ear)

  function: transmit vibrations from the external ear to the internal ear. The vibratory force of the tympanic membrane amplifies sound 15 times at the fenestra vestibuli

C. **Internal Ear:** consists of a series of canals in the petrous portion of the temporal bone. It consists of the outer bony labyrinth and an inner membranous labyrinth.

Refer to Figure 19.2 to identify the various parts of the bony and membranous labyrinth

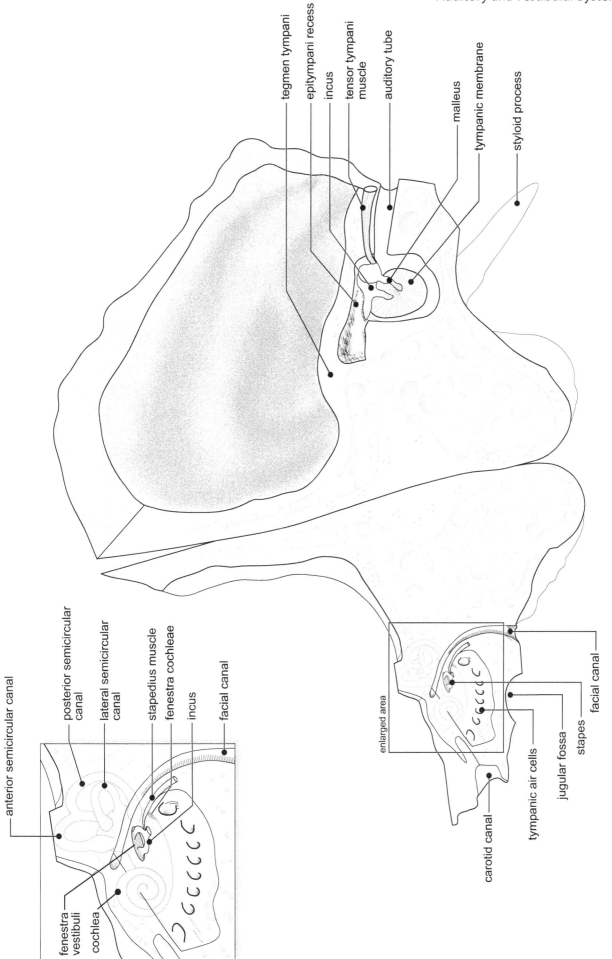

Figure 19.1   Structure of the middle and internal ear

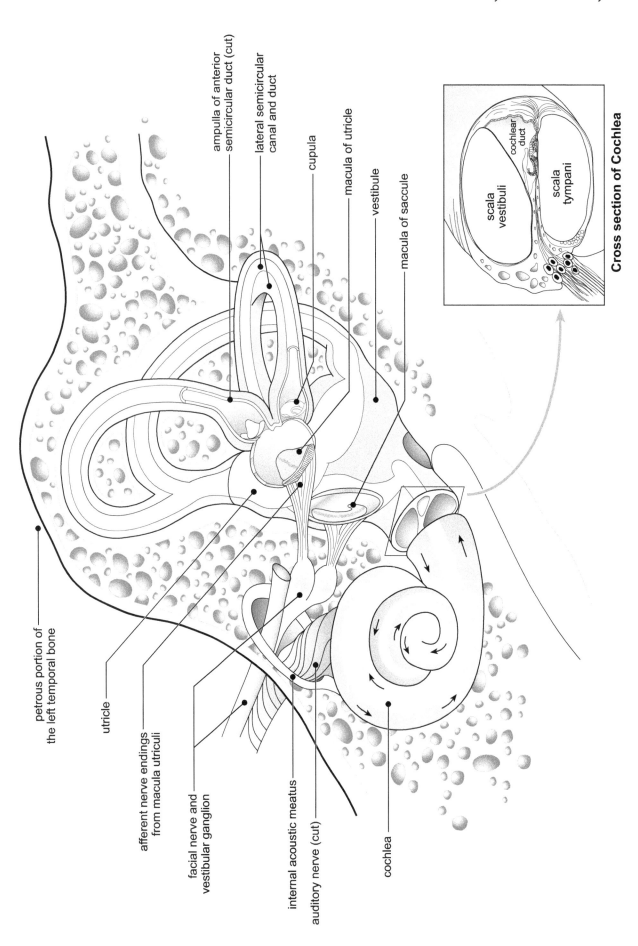

ampulla of anterior semicircular duct (cut)

lateral semicircular canal and duct

cupula

macula of utricle

vestibule

macula of saccule

Cross section of Cochlea

scala vestibuli

cochlear duct

scala tympani

petrous portion of the left temporal bone

utricle

afferent nerve endings from macula utriculi

facial nerve and vestibular ganglion

internal acoustic meatus

auditory nerve (cut)

cochlea

Figure 19.2   Structure of the internal ear

a. *Bony labyrinth*: contains *perilymph* (decreased K⁺; increased Na⁺ ions)

Consists of:

- **cochlea:** is the anteromedial portion of the bony labyrinth
- **vestibule:** is the central portion
- **semicircular canals:** extend posterolaterally from the vestibule and consists of the anterior, posterior and lateral semicircular canals

b. *Membranous labyrinth*: located within the bony labyrinth and contains *endolymph* (increased K⁺, decreased Na⁺ ions)

Consists of:

- *cochlear duct*: contained in the cochlea
- *utricle* and *saccule*: contained in the vestibule
- *semicircular ducts*: contained in the semicircular canals and arise from the utricle

i. **Cochlea**

- is a bony spiral canal that makes 2 and one-half turns around a bony core, the *modiolus*
- within the cavity of the modiolus is the *spiral ganglion.* Central processes of the bipolar neurons in the spiral ganglion form the *cochlear nerve;* peripheral processes innervate hair cells
- the interior of the cochlea is divided by the *vestibular* and *basilar membranes* into three compartments. Refer to Figure 19.2 to identify the three compartments in a cross section of the cochlea

These are:
  a. **scala vestibuli,** contains perilymph and is separated by the *vestibular membrane* from the scala media
  b. **scala media** or **cochlear duct**, contains endolymph and is separated by the *basilar membrane* from the scala tympani
  c. **scala tympani** contains perilymph

ii. *Cochlear duct or Scala media*:

The relationship of the following structures can be easily understood if the cochlea is visualized as having three compartments (Figure 19.2), the middle compartment is the cochlear duct. The cochlear duct is the membranous labyrinth, triangular in cross section, and filled with endolymph

An enlarged view of the basilar membrane and organ of Corti is indicated in Figure 19.3

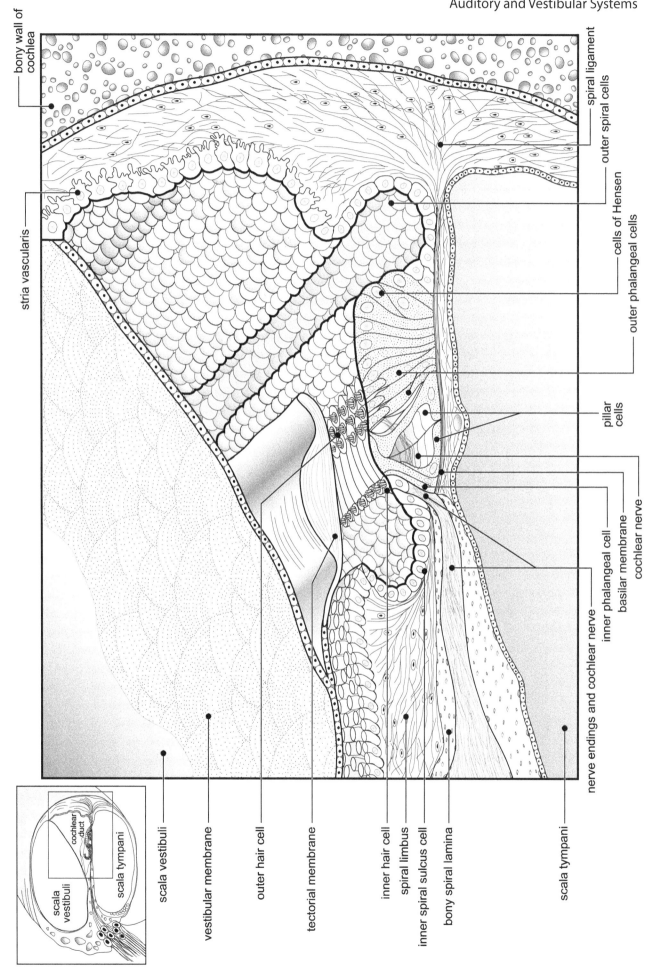

bony wall of cochlea

spiral ligament

outer spiral cells

cells of Hensen

outer phalangeal cells

stria vascularis

pillar cells

inner phalangeal cell

basilar membrane

cochlear nerve

nerve endings and cochlear nerve

scala vestibuli

vestibular membrane

outer hair cell

tectorial membrane

inner hair cell

spiral limbus

inner spiral sulcus cell

bony spiral lamina

scala tympani

scala vestibuli

cochlear duct

scala tympani

Figure 19.3   Structure of the cochlear duct and spiral organ of Corti

The cochlear duct consists of the following:

    a. ***basilar membrane***:
- is composed of collagen and elastic fibers
- on it rests the ***organ of Corti***
- is attached to the spiral lamina (at the modiolus) and the outer wall of the cochlear duct
- it increases in width from base to apex of cochlea
- high tones cause increase vibration of the basilar membrane at base of cochlea; low tones cause increase vibration at the apex of the cochlea

    b. **Organ of Corti** (spiral organ)
- rests on the basilar membrane
- consists of the following:
  - i. supporting cells of 1-5 rows
  - ii. sensory cells:
- consists of inner and outer hair cells (1-5 rows); 50 -150 hairs (microvilli) per cell
- hairs contact tectorial membrane, a glycoprotein layer that overhangs the *organ of Corti*
- vibration of the basilar membrane activates hair cells (from base to apex of cochlea) resulting in initiation of action potentials in the sensory nerve endings of sensory neurons in the spiral ganglion

    Clinical Notes:
- degenerative changes in the *organ of Corti* results in high tone deafness

iii. **Sound Transduction**:

Refer to Figure 19.2 to follow the sequence of events as described below.

Air pressure waves cause:
- vibration of tympanic membrane, slow vibration in response to low-pitched sounds or rapid vibration in response to high-pitched sounds

$\Rightarrow$ vibration of malleus, incus and stapes
$\Rightarrow$ displacement of fenestra vestibuli
$\Rightarrow$ resulting in vibration of the perilymph in scala vestibuli
$\Rightarrow$ vibration of vestibular membrane
$\Rightarrow$ vibration of endolymph in cochlear duct
$\Rightarrow$ vibration of basilar membrane
$\Rightarrow$ displacement of sensory cells, bending of hairs (microvilli) relative to the tectorial membrane
$\Rightarrow$ depolarization of sensory cells
$\Rightarrow$ action potentials generated via peripheral branches of sensory neurons in spiral ganglion

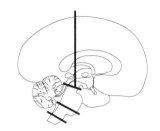

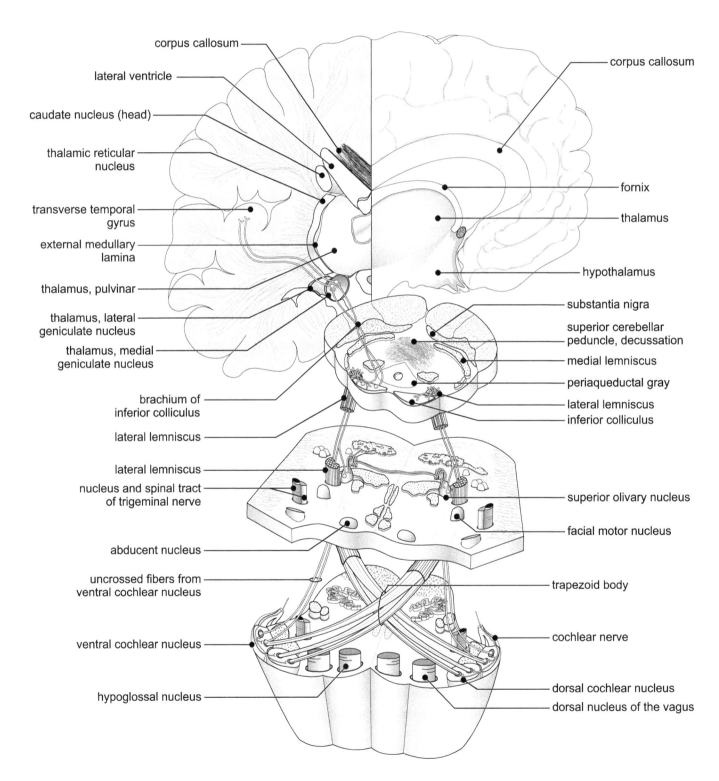

Figure 19.4   Central auditory pathways

IV. Central Auditory Pathways

Refer to Figure 19.4 for details of the central auditory pathways. The ascending pathway consists of sequence of neurons that are arranged as follows:

- central processes of neurons in the spiral ganglion form the ***cochlear nerve***

  ⇒ pass through internal auditory meatus
  ⇒ enter at the brain stem at the cerebellopontine angle
  ⇒ synapse in ***dorsal cochlear nucleus*** and ***ventral cochlear nucleus,*** at base of inferior cerebellar peduncle
  ⇒ fibers from the dorsal and ventral cochlear nuclei cross the midline in the tegmentum of the pons, forming the ***trapezoid body***. Fibers from the ventral cochlear nucleus either synapse in the ipsilateral or contralateral ***superior olivary nucleus*** or continue rostrally to join the ***lateral lemniscus***. Some fibers from the cochlear nuclei do not cross the midline and continue rostrally in the ipsilateral lateral lemniscus. Each lateral lemniscus carries information from both ears.
  ⇒ lateral lemniscus terminates in the ***inferior colliculus***
  ⇒ fibers from the inferior colliculus constitute the ***inferior brachium***
  ⇒ terminates in the ***medial geniculate nucleus***
  ⇒ via the ***auditory radiation*** in the internal capsule
  ⇒ to ***primary auditory area*** of the temporal lobe
      anterolateral area = low tones
      posteromedial area = high tones

VESTIBULAR SYSTEM

Overview

The vestibular system is important in orientation of the head in space and in controlling eye movements with respect to maintaining balance. The sensory receptors are located in the membranous labyrinth of the internal ear (Figure 19.2).

I. Anatomy of the Membranous Labyrinth

a. ***Utricle*** and ***Saccule*** are enclosed in the vestibule of the bony labyrinth (Figure 19.2) and constitutes the ***static labyrinth.***

   The static labyrinth functions in maintaining the position of the head relative to the force of gravity.

b. ***Semicircular ducts*** (3) are enclosed in each of the three semicircular canals of the bony labyrinth (Figure 19.2) and constitutes the ***kinetic labyrinth***.

   The kinetic labyrinth detects movements of the head.

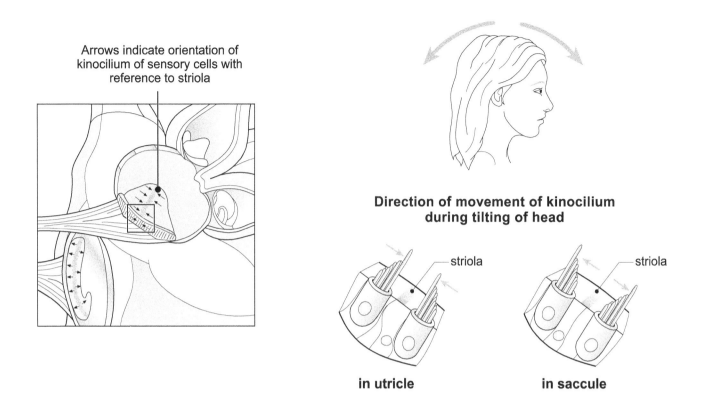

Arrows indicate orientation of kinocilium of sensory cells with reference to striola

Direction of movement of kinocilium during tilting of head

striola

striola

in utricle

in saccule

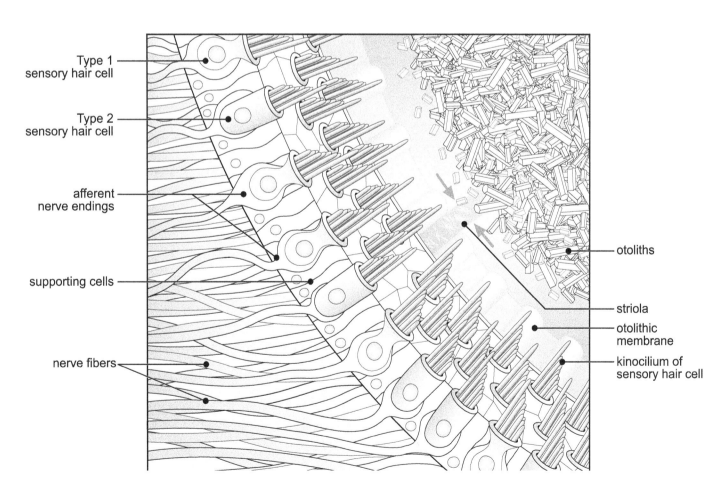

Type 1 sensory hair cell

Type 2 sensory hair cell

afferent nerve endings

supporting cells

nerve fibers

otoliths

striola

otolithic membrane

kinocilium of sensory hair cell

Figure 19.5   Structure of the macula in utricle

A. **Static labyrinth**

Receptors are located in the utricle and saccule and called *macula* (Figures 19.2 and 19.5)

   i. *macula utriculi* are receptors in the utricle
       * is located on the floor of the utricle
       * is horizontally placed
       * responds when head is flexed or extended

   ii. *macula sacculi* are receptors in the saccule
       * is located on the medial wall
       * is vertically placed
       * responds when head is tilted to one side

Structure of maculae utriculi and sacculi (Figure 19.5):

Consists of:

* *supporting cells*
* *sensory hair cell*s are of two types. Type 1 cell is flask-shaped and Type 2 cell is cylindrical (Figure 19.5). Each sensory cell consists of:
    * 30-50 *stereocilia* (large microvilli) and a long cilium, the ***kinocilium***
    * in the macula utriculi, kinocilia of hair cells are oriented with respect to a central line, the *striola (*Figure 19.5). In the macula sacculi, kinocilia face away from the *striola.* Thus, different areas along the macula are specialized to detect movement in a particular direction.
    * hairs are embedded in an ***otolithic membrane***, which contain otoliths (concretions of calcium carbonate)
* if the head is tilted, gravitational force on the otoliths cause displacement of the hairs causing bending of hairs towards the kinocilium, resulting in depolarization of sensory cells
* impulses are carried by the peripheral branches of the bipolar neurons located in the ***vestibular ganglion***, at the internal auditory meatus.

B. **Kinetic labyrinth**

Includes three ***semicircular ducts***. These are ***anterior***, ***posterior*** and ***lateral semicircular ducts*** (Figure 19.2). The three semicircular ducts are arranged as a functional pair and lie in same plane. For example, when the head is in the upright position, the anterior and posterior canals are in the vertical plane, whereas the lateral canals are in the horizontal plane.

Structure of Crista ampullaris:

Refer to Figure 19.6 for the structural features of the crista ampullaris

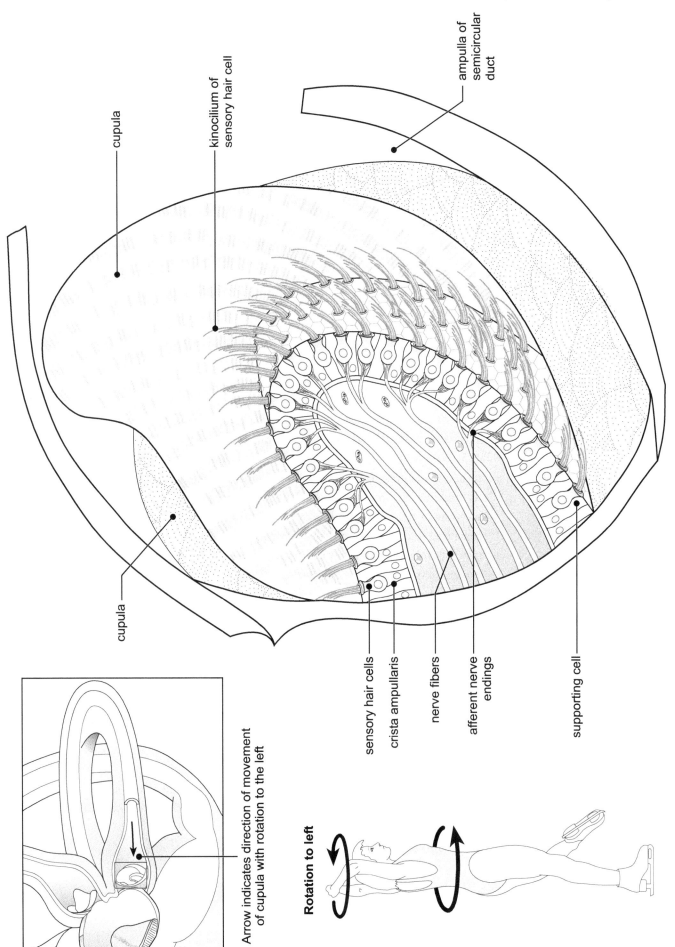

cupula

kinocilium of
sensory hair cell

ampulla of
semicircular
duct

cupula

sensory hair cells

crista ampullaris

nerve fibers

afferent nerve
endings

supporting cell

Arrow indicates direction of movement
of cupula with rotation to the left

Rotation to left

Figure 19.6   Structure of the crista ampullaris

- each semicircular duct has an expansion at one of its end, the *ampulla,* which opens into the utricle.
- each ampulla consists of a ridge of sensory epithelium, the *crista ampullaris.*
- the crista ampullaris consists of *supporting cells* and *sensory hair cells.*

- each sensory cell consists of:
    - *stereocilia* and a *kinocilium*
    - the stereocilia and kinocilium are embedded in a gelatinous material that lacks otoliths and called *cupula.* The cupula is dome-shaped and extends upward into the ampulla.

- rotating the head to the left causes the endolymph in the right lateral semicircular duct to lag behind, due to inertia. This delay results in backward flow of endolymph in the right lateral semicircular duct and displacement of the cupula and stereocilia of sensory cells away from the utricle, resulting in hyperpolarization of the sensory cells of the right lateral semicircular duct. Bending and stimulation of the sensory cells is interpreted as rotation to the left.
- impulses are carried by the peripheral branches of the bipolar neurons in the *vestibular ganglion*, which is located at the internal auditory meatus.
Central branches of bipolar neurons join the vestibulocochlear nerve

II. Central pathways

A. *Vestibular nuclei* are located in the rostral medulla and caudal pons, beneath the lateral part of the floor of the fourth ventricle

The four nuclei are: *lateral*, *superior*, *medial* and *inferior vestibular nuclei*

i) *Afferents to the vestibular nuclei are*:

- vestibular nerve
- cerebellovestibular fibers

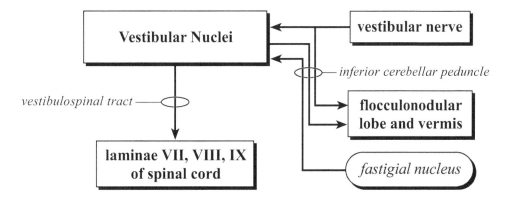

Figure 19.7   Schematic diagram of connections of the vestibular nuclei

function: excitatory to extensors of ipsilateral lower limb, flexors are inhibited thereby regulating muscle tone with reference to posture and balance

ii) *Efferents from the vestibular nuclei are*:

    a. **lateral vestibulospinal tract**

- maculae
  ⇓
  lateral vestibular nucleus
  ⇓ (uncrossed)
  laminae VII, VIII, IX of cervical and lumbosacral enlargements of the cord

function: excitatory to extensors of trunk and limbs

    b. **Medial vestibulospinal tract**

- maculae
  ⇓
  medial vestibular nucleus
  ⇓
  cervical and thoracic segments of spinal cord

function: head movements for balance and fixation of gaze

    c. **Medial longitudinal fasciculus**

- crista
  ⇓
  medial vestibular nucleus
  ⇓
  medial longitudinal fasciculus
  ⇓
  nuclei of oculomotor, trochlear and abducent nerves

function: coordinated movements of eyes and head (vestibulo-ocular reflex)

Clinical Notes:

i. lesion of the vestibular nerve causes nausea, nystagmus; vertigo
ii. **Meniere's disease** is caused by overproduction of endolymph in membranous labyrinth, symptoms are vertigo (false sense of rotation) and loss of hearing

CHAPTER
20

VENTRICLES, MENINGES AND BLOOD SUPPLY

Overview

Ventricles are cavities in the brain and spinal cord that contain cerebrospinal fluid. Ventricles are lined by ependyma and communicate with each other and with the subarachnoid space through apertures.

I. Ventricles

The cavities of the brain consist of a pair of **lateral ventricles**, the **third ventricle**, the **cerebral aqueduct** and the **fourth ventricle**, which in turn is connected to the subarachnoid space and the **central canal** of the spinal cord (Figure 20.1). Many of the ventricles have been described previously, only the lateral ventricles will be described in this section

Lateral ventricles

The largest ventricles, the lateral ventricles are C-shaped cavities in each of the cerebral hemispheres. Lateral ventricles are lined by ependyma, where it is invaginated by the pia mater to form the **choroid plexus.** The lateral ventricles are connected to the third ventricle through the **interventricular foramen**. Each ventricle consists of the following parts. These are: **frontal horn**, **central part**, **collateral trigone**, **temporal horn** and **occipital horn**.

A. Parts of the Lateral Ventricle:

Refer to Figure 20.1 for the various parts of the lateral ventricle. These are:

i. **Frontal horn**: extends anteriorly from the interventricular foramen into frontal lobe. The **interventricular foramen** at junction of the fornix and anterior nucleus of the thalamus connects the lateral ventricle to the third ventricle

- in sections of the brain, the major boundaries of the frontal horn are as follows:

  roof: corpus callosum (genu)
  medial wall: septum pellucidum
  lateral wall: caudate nucleus (head)

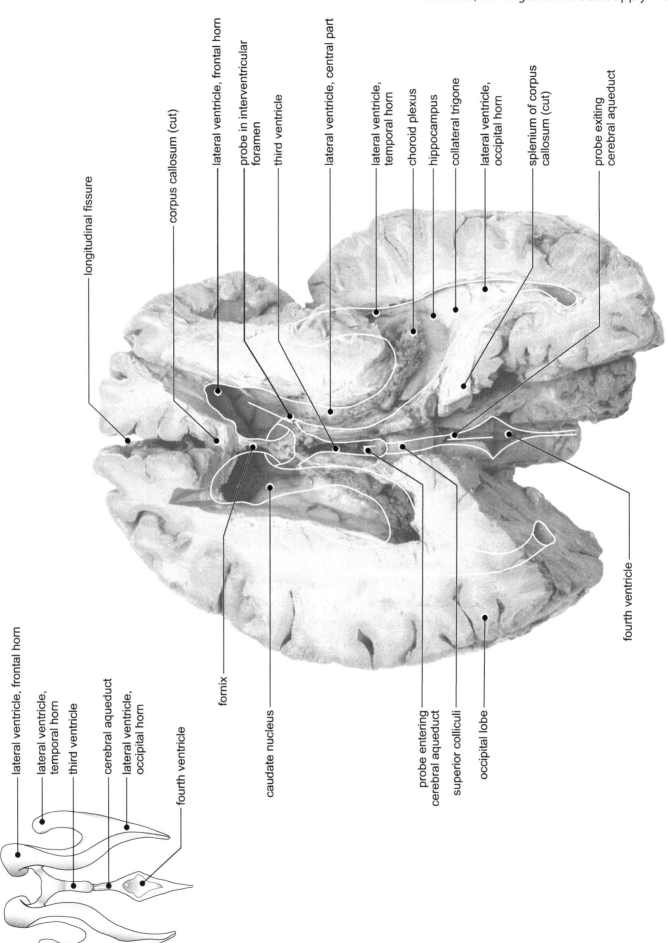

longitudinal fissure

corpus callosum (cut)

lateral ventricle, frontal horn

probe in interventricular foramen

third ventricle

lateral ventricle, central part

lateral ventricle, temporal horn

choroid plexus

hippocampus

collateral trigone

lateral ventricle, occipital horn

splenium of corpus callosum (cut)

probe exiting cerebral aqueduct

fornix

caudate nucleus

probe entering cerebral aqueduct

superior colliculi

occipital lobe

fourth ventricle

lateral ventricle, frontal horn

lateral ventricle, temporal horn

third ventricle

cerebral aqueduct

lateral ventricle, occipital horn

fourth ventricle

Figure 20.1   Dissection of the ventricles of the brain

ii. ***Central part*** (***body***): is located in the area of the parietal lobe

   roof: is formed by the corpus callosum
   floor: is formed by the thalamus (dorsal surface) and fornix

iii. ***Collateral trigone***: is a triangular area, located at the junction of the central part (body), temporal horn and occipital horn

iv. ***Temporal horn***: is located in the temporal lobe

   • in sections, the boundaries are as follows:

   roof: tail of caudate nucleus
   floor: hippocampus

v. ***Occipital horn***: is located in the occipital lobe (Figure 17.1)

   On the *medial wall* is the:
   • forceps major forms an impression, referred to as the ***bulb of occipital horn***
   • the calcarine sulcus forms an impression, referred to as the ***calcar avis***

B. Choroid Plexus and Cerebrospinal fluid:

Cerebrospinal fluid circulates in the ventricles of the brain and the central canal of the spinal cord. Cerebrospinal fluid is produced by the choroid plexus and drained via the arachnoid villi into the dural venous sinuses.

i. ***Choroid plexus***:

   • are vascular folds of pia mater and ependyma (Figure 20.1)
   • composed of a core of connective tissue layer covered by a layer of cuboidal epithelium
   • the connective tissue contains an extensive network of fenestrated capillaries
   • tight junctions between cells prevent passage of macromolecules from blood vessels into CSF, constituting the ***blood-CSF barrier***

ii. ***Cerebrospinal fluid:***

   a. ***General features***:

   • secreted by the epithelial cells that line the ***choroid plexus*** in the lateral ventricles, third ventricle and fourth ventricles
   • 80-140 ml of cerebrospinal fluid are contained in the ventricles and subarachnoid space

- is a colorless, ultrafiltrate of plasma with little protein, glucose, few lymphocytes and large amounts of sodium chloride
- CSF production involves active transport of Na^+ and ions and passive diffusion of water

b. *Circulation of cerebrospinal fluid*:

- cerebrospinal fluid (CSF) flows from the *lateral ventricles* into the *third ventricle* through two openings, the *interventricular foramina* (Figure 20.1).
- the fluid then flows through the **cerebral aqueduct** into the *fourth ventricle*.
- CSF enters the subarachnoid space through the *median aperture* and the paired *lateral apertures*, which then circulates in the *subarachnoid space* and *central canal of the spinal cord*.
- CSF is gradually reabsorbed into the venous blood through **arachnoid villi** into the **superior sagittal sinus** (Figure 20.3). Absorption is dependent on the pressure gradient between CSF, arterial blood and venous blood. Arachnoid villi become hypertrophied with age and are then referred to as *arachnoid granulations*
- circulation of CSF is unidirectional and is assisted by the pulsation of arteries in the subarachnoid space

C. Functions of cerebrospinal fluid

- cushions the brain and absorbs forces
- maintains chemical environment for neuronal signalling
- circulates nutrients and removes waste products

Clinical Notes:
Tumors, inflammation can obstruct the drainage of cerebrospinal fluid (CSF). When excess cerebrospinal fluid accumulates in the ventricles, CSF pressure rises and this condition is referred to as *hydrocephalus*.

Types of hydrocephalus:

i. *External hydrocephalus*: atrophy of the brain results in excess CSF in subarachnoid space eg. senile atrophy
ii. *Internal hydrocephalus*: is dilation of ventricles, due to obstruction of fourth ventricle or cerebral aqueduct
iii. *Communicating hydrocephalus*: is a combination of external and internal hydrocephalus and is due to an obstruction of arachnoid villi caused by a subarachnoid hemorrhage.

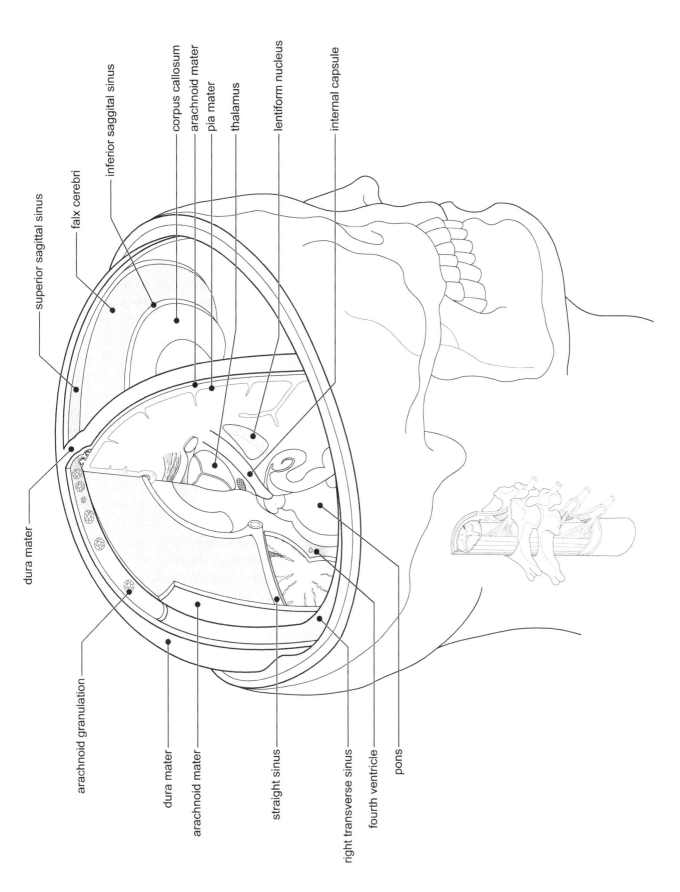

superior sagittal sinus

falx cerebri

inferior saggital sinus

corpus callosum

arachnoid mater

pia mater

thalamus

lentiform nucleus

internal capsule

dura mater

arachnoid granulation

dura mater

arachnoid mater

straight sinus

right transverse sinus

fourth ventricle

pons

Figure 20.2   Meninges of the brain

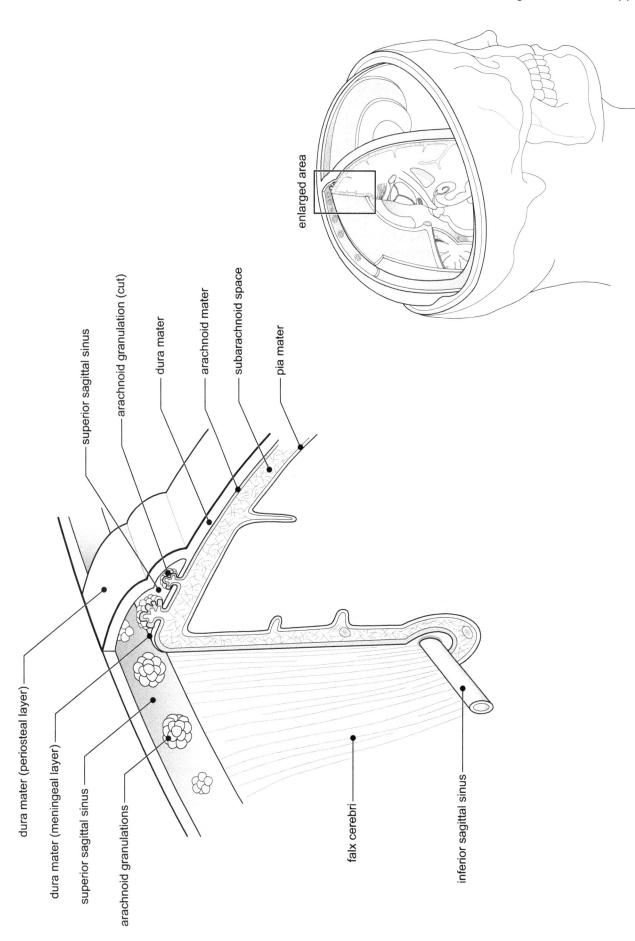

dura mater (periosteal layer)

dura mater (meningeal layer)

superior sagittal sinus

arachnoid granulations

superior sagittal sinus

arachnoid granulation (cut)

dura mater

arachnoid mater

subarachnoid space

pia mater

falx cerebri

inferior sagittal sinus

enlarged area

Figure 20.3   Enlarged view of the meninges of the brain

II. Meninges

Overview

The meninges consist of three layers of connective tissue that cover the brain and spinal cord. The layers are the outer dura mater, the arachnoid mater deep to the dura mater and the innermost pia mater. The dura mater supports the brain and spinal cord and provides protection from the skull and vertebral column that contain them.

A. Dura mater:

- is the outer covering of dense connective tissue and is attached with the periosteum of the skull
- it is separated from the arachnoid mater by the ***subdural space***
- it folds to form four partitions or processes in several regions of the skull
- ***dural venous sinuses*** are located between the periosteum and the dura mater and along areas of attachment of the partitions (Figures 20.2 and 20.3)

1. ***Processes of the dura mater***:

    Separates parts of the brain and are indicated in Figure 20.4. These are:

    i. *falx cerebri*:
        - is located in the longitudinal fissure, between the cerebral hemispheres
        - it attaches from the crista galli to the internal occipital protuberance and superior surface of tentorium cerebelli
    ii. ***tentorium cerebelli***:
        - is located between occipital lobes of the cerebrum and cerebellum
        - it attaches at the superior border of petrous portion of temporal bones and margins of the groove for the transverse sinuses
    iii. *falx cerebelli*:
        - is located between the cerebellar hemispheres
    iv. ***diaphragma sellae***:
        - forms roof over pituitary gland

2. **Dural venous sinuses**

    The locations of the dural venous sinuses are indicated in Figure 20.4. The following dural venous sinuses are:

    i. ***superior sagittal sinus:***
        - is located along the superior border of the falx cerebri
        - is continuous with the right transverse sinus

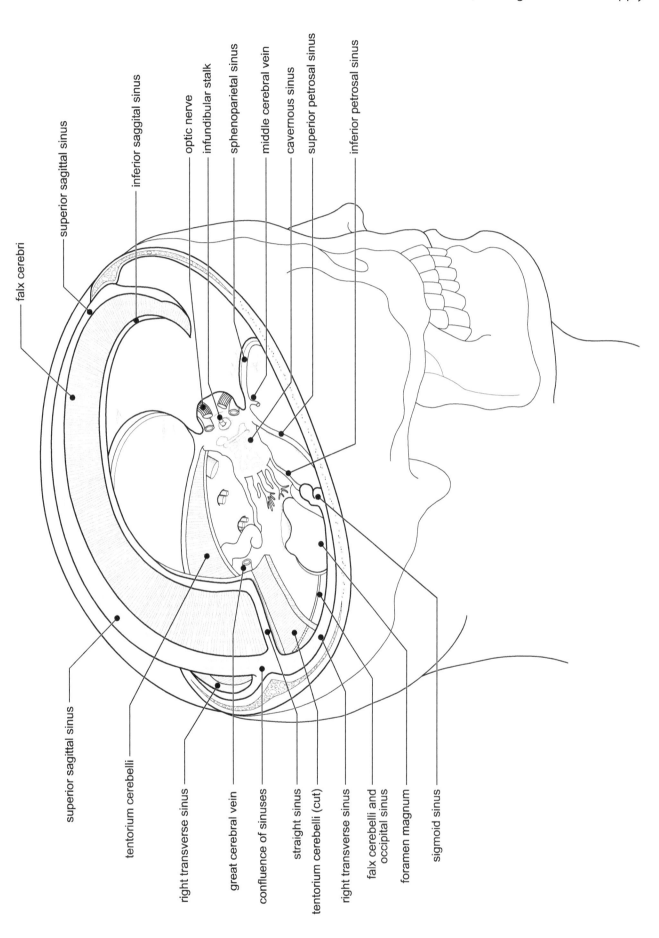

falx cerebri

superior sagittal sinus

inferior saggital sinus

optic nerve

infundibular stalk

sphenoparietal sinus

middle cerebral vein

cavernous sinus

superior petrosal sinus

inferior petrosal sinus

superior sagittal sinus

tentorium cerebelli

right transverse sinus

great cerebral vein

confluence of sinuses

straight sinus

tentorium cerebelli (cut)

right transverse sinus

falx cerebelli and occipital sinus

foramen magnum

sigmoid sinus

Figure 20.4   Dural processes and dural venous sinuses

    ii. *inferior sagittal sinus:*
- is located along the inferior border of the falx cerebri
- drains into the straight sinus

    iii. *straight sinus:*
- located at the attachment of the falx cerebri and tentorium cerebelli
- receives the *great cerebral vein*
- continuous with the left transverse sinus

    iv. *confluence of sinuses:*
- located at internal occipital protuberance
- it is formed by connections of the straight sinus, right and left transverse sinuses and occipital sinus.

    v. *occipital sinus:*
- located in the attached margin of the falx cerebelli

    vi. *transverse sinuses:*
- each sinus is located in a groove on the occipital bone, along the attached margin of the tentorium cerebelli
- is continuous with the sigmoid sinuses

    vii. *sigmoid sinuses*:
- each sinus is located at the petrous portion of the temporal bone
- is continuous with the internal jugular vein

3. **Arachnoid mater:**

- is a thin, middle fibrous layer (Figures 20.2 and 20.3)
- numerous trabeculae extend from the arachnoid mater to the pia mater
- projections of arachnoid mater form the ***arachnoid villi***
- the ***subarachnoid space***, containing ***cerebrospinal fluid***, is located between the arachnoid mater and the pia mater

4. **Pia mater**:

- is a thin fibrous innermost layer; dips into sulci (Figure 20.3) and carries blood vessels to deeper layers

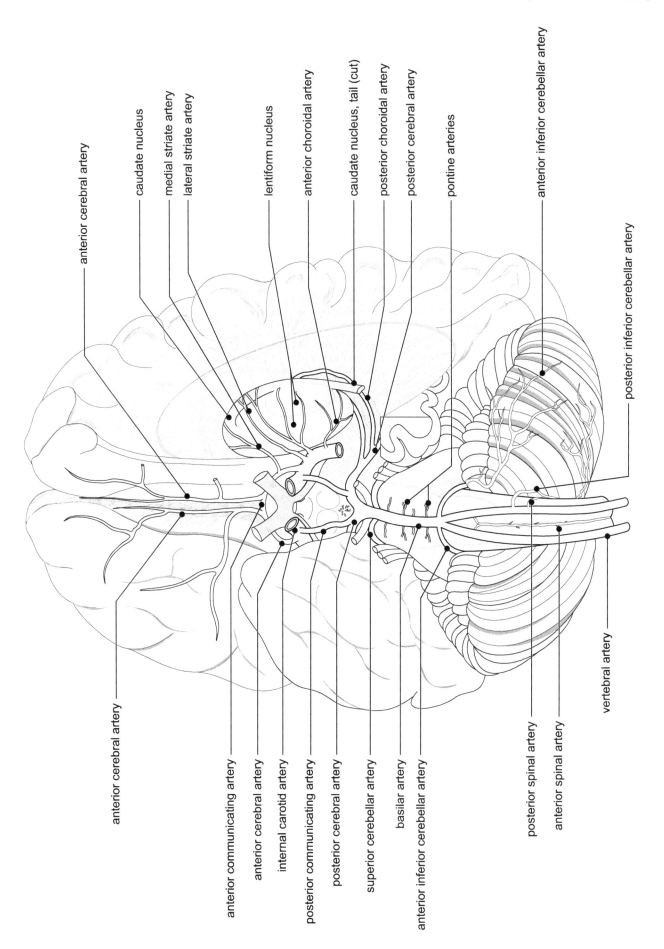

anterior cerebral artery

caudate nucleus

medial striate artery

lateral striate artery

lentiform nucleus

anterior choroidal artery

caudate nucleus, tail (cut)

posterior choroidal artery

posterior cerebral artery

pontine arteries

anterior inferior cerebellar artery

posterior inferior cerebellar artery

anterior cerebral artery

anterior communicating artery

anterior cerebral artery

internal carotid artery

posterior communicating artery

posterior cerebral artery

superior cerebellar artery

basilar artery

anterior inferior cerebellar artery

posterior spinal artery

anterior spinal artery

vertebral artery

Figure 20.5   Blood supply of the brain

III. Blood Supply (Arterial Supply)

The brain comprises only 2% of the body weight, however, it receives 17% of the cardiac output and consumes about 20% of oxygen used by the entire body. The brain requires a rich blood supply. Loss of blood supply for more than a few minutes results in irreversible brain damage and unconsciousness occurs if the blood supply is interrupted for few seconds. Cerebrovascular lesions constitute the major cause of neurological disorders.

Major Arteries of the Brain:

The brain is supplied by the *internal carotid* and *vertebral arteries*

A. Internal carotid artery:

Courses through the neck, passes through the carotid canal, enters the cranial cavity and divides into the *anterior cerebral* and *middle cerebral arteries* lateral to the optic chiasm (Figures 8.4 and 20.5)

Branches:
- *ophthalmic artery* – supplies the orbit
- *hypophyseal artery* – supplies the hypophysis
- *anterior choroidal artery* – is a long thin artery and frequently involved in cerebrovascular disorders. It supplies the hippocampus; amygdala; uncus; globus pallidus; thalamus, subthalamus, optic tract
- *posterior communicating artery* – joins posterior cerebral artery to complete the Circle of Willis

Clinical Notes:
    Internal carotid artery occlusion causes:
- blindness in ipsilateral eye
- contralateral homonymous hemianopia (if optic tract is involved)

B. Middle cerebral artery:

- runs laterally into the lateral sulcus and divides into many branches to supply the lateral surface of frontal, parietal and temporal lobes (Figure 20.6)

    Note: includes motor, sensory, auditory and speech areas

Branches:
- *lateral striate artery* (anterolateral group):
  supplies the caudate nucleus; putamen; pallidum; internal capsule; external capsule and claustrum

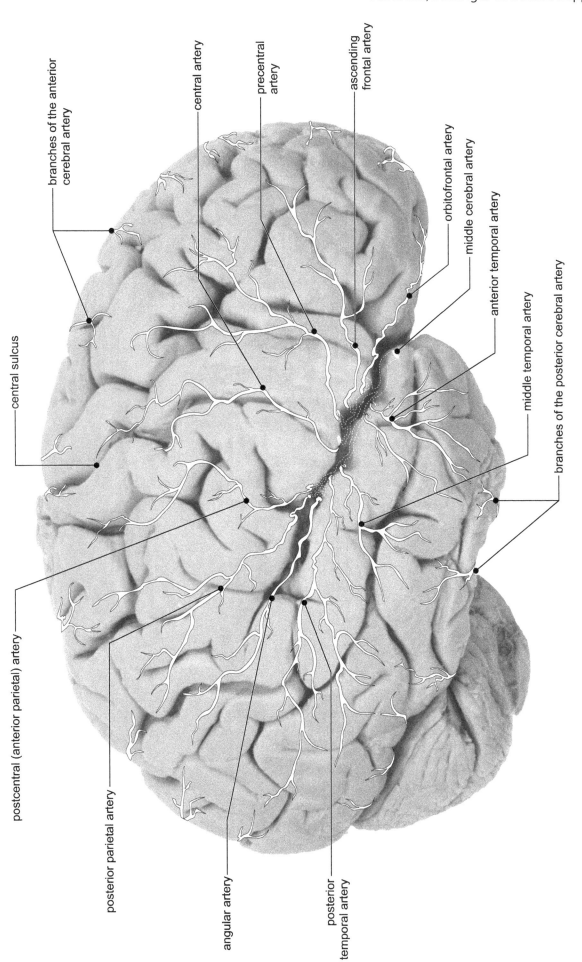

branches of the anterior cerebral artery

central artery

precentral artery

ascending frontal artery

orbitofrontal artery

middle cerebral artery

anterior temporal artery

middle temporal artery

branches of the posterior cerebral artery

central sulcus

postcentral (anterior parietal) artery

posterior parietal artery

angular artery

posterior temporal artery

Figure 20.6   Distribution of the middle cerebral artery on the lateral surface of the cerebral hemisphere

Clinical Notes:

Middle cerebral artery occlusion causes:

- contralateral hemiplegia
- hemisensory deficits
- homonymous hemianopia
- global aphasia (left hemisphere)

C. Anterior cerebral artery:

- runs superior and medially towards the longitudinal fissure and is joined with the artery of the opposite side by the ***anterior communicating artery***
- it supplies the medial surfaces of frontal and parietal lobes and the olfactory tract (Figure 20.7)

Branches:

- ***recurrent artery of Heubner*** (***medial striate artery***): supplies caudate, putamen and internal capsule

Clinical Notes:

Anterior cerebral artery occlusion causes:

- contralateral motor and sensory deficits – leg and perineum (pelvic floor)
- ipsilateral anosmia
- contralateral upper motor neuron weakness of face and tongue (if involves genu of internal capsule)

D. Posterior cerebral artery:

- the artery curves around the midbrain and divides into many branches to supply the temporal lobe and occipital lobe (Figure 20.7)

Branches:

- ***posterior choroidal artery***: supplies thalamus; fornix; midbrain

Clinical Notes:

Posterior cerebral artery occlusion causes:

- homonymous hemianopia
- alexia (if involves splenium of corpus callosum)
- memory loss (if bilateral)

E. Basilar artery:

- the artery lies on the basilar sulcus of the pons
- terminates into the posterior cerebral arteries

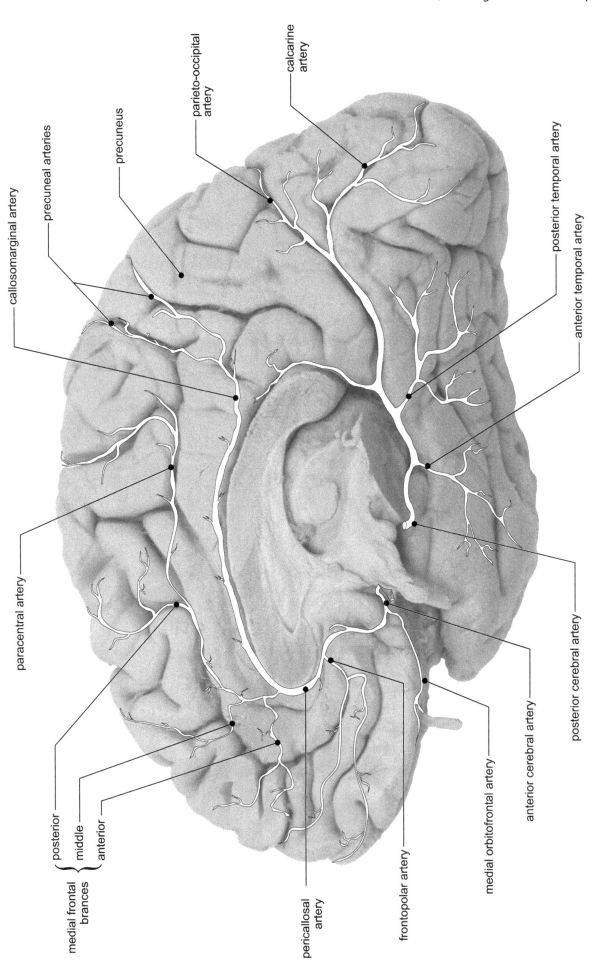

calcarine artery

parieto-occipital artery

precuneus

precuneal arteries

callosomarginal artery

posterior temporal artery

anterior temporal artery

paracentral artery

posterior
middle
anterior
} medial frontal brances

pericallosal artery

frontopolar artery

medial orbitofrontal artery

anterior cerebral artery

posterior cerebral artery

Figure 20.7   Distribution of the anterior and posterior cerebral arteries on the medial surface of the cerebral hemisphere

Branches:
- ***superior cerebellar artery*** and ***anterior inferior cerebellar artery*** "AICA".
  It supplies the cerebellum, pons and medulla

F. Vertebral artery:

- the two vertebral arteries join at the caudal border of the pons to form the basilar
  artery

Branches:

- ***posterior inferior cerebellar artery*** "PICA" supplies the cerebellum and
  medulla
- ***anterior spinal artery***: supplies the ventral and dorsal gray horns; ventral
  and lateral funiculi of spinal cord
- ***posterior spinal artery***: of spinal cord supplies dorsal gray horn and dorsal
  funiculi

Additional branches to the spinal cord are from:

Segmental spinal arteries that arise from the intercostal arteries and the abdominal aorta.

These are :
- **anterior and posterior radicular arteries:** supplies the lower cervical,
  thoracic, lumbar and sacral regions of the spinal cord

G. Circle of Willis

1. ***Formation:***

   formed by the anterior cerebral arteries, anterior communicating artery, internal
   carotid arteries, posterior communicating arteries, posterior cerebral arteries

   Significance – provides an alternate route of circulation in case of occlusion of a
   major artery

2. Four groups of ***central arteries*** arise from the ***Circle of Willis***.

   These are:
   - ***a. Anteromedial group***: supplies the hypothalamus
   - ***b. Anterolateral group*** (***lateral striate artery***): supplies the caudate nucleus;
     putamen; pallidum; internal capsule; external capsule and claustrum
   - ***c. Posteromedial group***: supplies the thalamus; subthalamus; hypothalamus;
     cerebral peduncle
   - ***d. Posterolateral group***: supplies the midbrain, thalamus; cerebral peduncle

CHAPTER
21

AUTONOMIC NERVOUS SYSTEM

Overview

The Autonomic Nervous System is a division of the peripheral nervous system and operates under involuntary control. It is comprised of ganglia and nerves that are concerned with efferent innervation of the viscera. Motor neurons (general visceral motor neurons) of the autonomic nervous system convey information from the central nervous system to supply smooth muscle, cardiac muscle and glands. Associated with efferent fibers of the autonomic system are afferents fibers from the viscera. Afferents fibers convey information from the internal organs to the central nervous system, cell bodies of sensory neurons (general visceral afferent neurons) are within the sensory ganglia of associated cranial or spinal nerves.   The autonomic nervous system consists of three parts, the sympathetic nervous system, the parasympathetic nervous system and the enteric nervous system. The sympathetic and parasympathetic nervous systems have antagonistic effects and are involved in the maintenance of homeostasis. Most organs are innervated by both systems. The sympathetic division increases the activity of the body during stressful situations as in a flight or fight response. The parasympathetic division decreases the activity of the body as in a relaxed state.   The enteric nervous system consists of hundred billion neurons located in the gastrointestinal tract that control secretions and contractions of the digestive tract.

I. Anatomy of the Autonomic Nervous System

The Autonomic Nervous System consists of two types of neurons:

1. **General visceral sensory neurons** transmit information from *chemoreceptors* that convey sensations such as feeling of fullness
2. **General visceral motor neurons** innervate *cardiac muscle, smooth muscle* and *glands.*

A. Autonomic Motor neurons

Motor neurons of the autonomic nervous system consists of a *chain of two neurons in succession* (Figure 21.1).

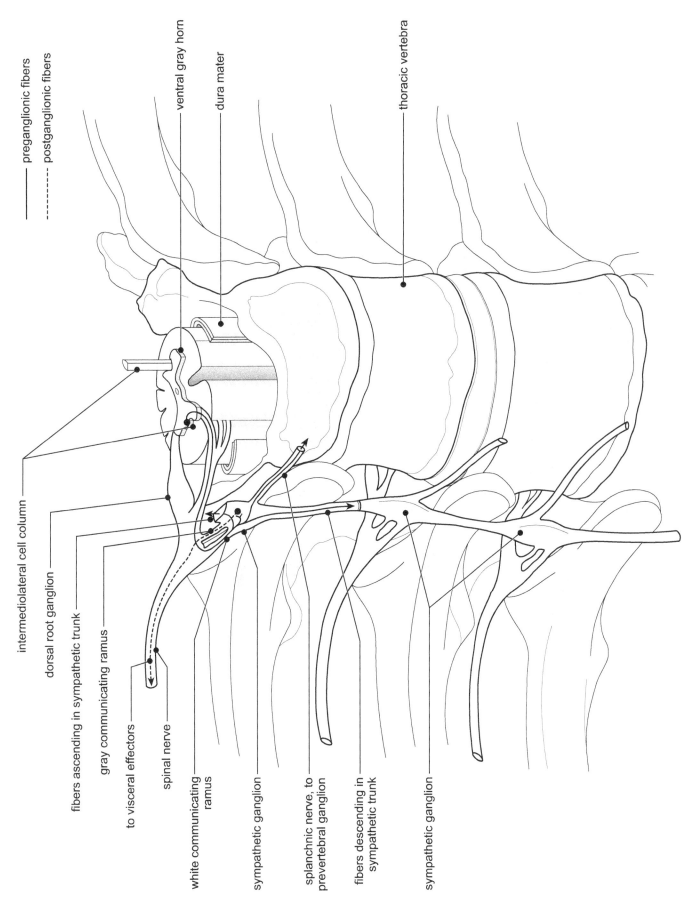

preganglionic fibers

postganglionic fibers

ventral gray horn

dura mater

thoracic vertebra

intermediolateral cell column

dorsal root ganglion

fibers ascending in sympathetic trunk

gray communicating ramus

to visceral effectors

spinal nerve

white communicating ramus

sympathetic ganglion

splanchnic nerve, to prevertebral ganglion

fibers descending in sympathetic trunk

sympathetic ganglion

Figure 21.1 Visceral efferent pathway of the Sympathetic Nervous System

1. The first motor neuron is referred to as the ***preganglionic neuron***

- its cell body is located in the brainstem or the spinal cord
- its axon, referred to as a ***preganglionic fiber***, exits the brain as part of a cranial or spinal nerve and terminates on a postganglionic neuron in an ***autonomic ganglion***
- each preganglionic fiber of the sympathetic system divides into many branches and synapses with multiple postganglionic neurons, therefore sympathetic effects have a widespread response throughout the body
- preganglionic sympathetic axons are short, preganglionic parasympathetic axons are long

2. The second motor neuron is referred to as the ***postganglionic neuron***

- its cell body is located in an autonomic ganglion
- its axon, referred to as a ***postganglionic fiber***, terminates by supplying a visceral effector
- parasympathetic preganglionic fibers synapse with four or five ***terminal ganglia*** that innervate a single visceral effector, therefore parasympathetic effects are localized
- postganglionic sympathetic axons are long, postganglionic parasympathetic axons are short

II. Organization and Location of the Sympathetic and Parasympathetic Autonomic Ganglia

A. Sympathetic Division

Consists of the following:

i. cell bodies of neurons located in the ***thoracic segments*** and ***upper lumbar segments*** of the spinal cord (Figure 21.2)

ii. ***Sympathetic trunks*** (Figure 21.2):

- are located on each side of the vertebral column that extend from the base of the skull to the coccyx
- are composed of nerves and series of ***ganglia***, referred to as ***paravertebral ganglia***. There are 3 *cervical*, 11 or 12 *thoracic*, 4 or 5 *lumbar* and 4 or 5 *sacral* autonomic ganglia.
- one paravertebral ganglion is associated with each spinal nerve, except at the cervical level where each sympathetic trunk consists of only three cervical ganglia as opposed to the eight cervical nerves.

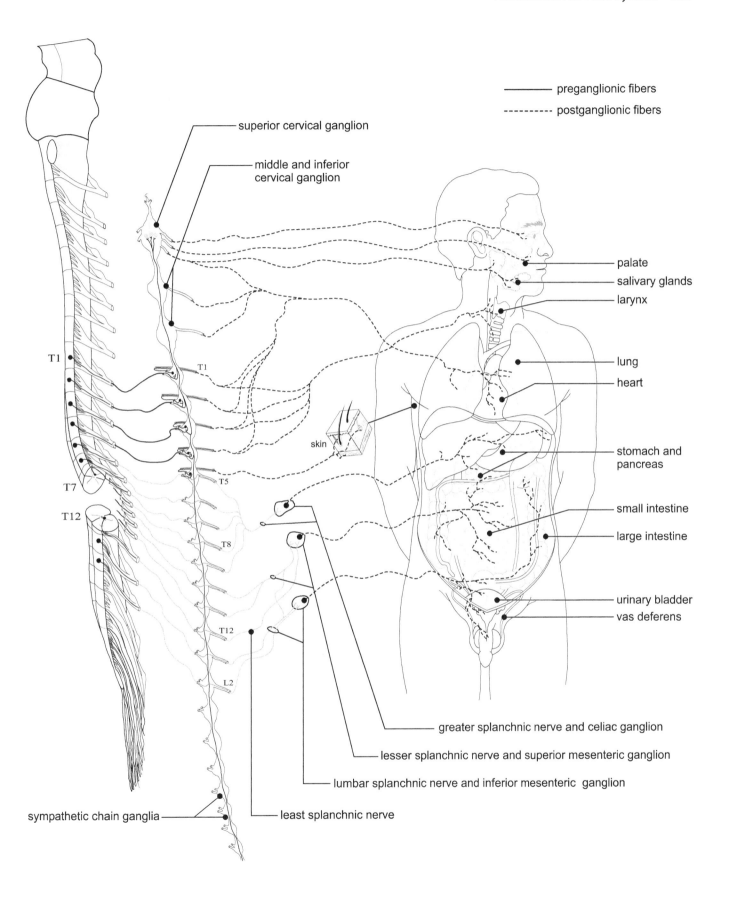

superior cervical ganglion

middle and inferior
cervical ganglion

preganglionic fibers

postganglionic fibers

palate

salivary glands

larynx

lung

heart

skin

stomach and
pancreas

small intestine

large intestine

urinary bladder

vas deferens

T1

T1

T7

T5

T12

T8

T12

L2

greater splanchnic nerve and celiac ganglion

lesser splanchnic nerve and superior mesenteric ganglion

lumbar splanchnic nerve and inferior mesenteric ganglion

sympathetic chain ganglia

least splanchnic nerve

Figure 21.2 Sympathetic Nervous System

iii. *Prevertebral (collateral) ganglia:*

- are located anterior to the vertebral column and in relation to the major blood vessels of the abdomen and pelvis
- preganglionic sympathetic fibers that do not synapse in the sympathetic ganglion and exit through the sympathetic trunk synapses in the prevertebral ganglia

B. Parasympathetic Ganglia (Figure 21.3)

Consists of the following:

i. cell bodies of neurons located in the brainstem and associated with ganglia of the *oculomotor*, *facial*, *glossopharyngeal* and *vagus* nerves

ii. cell bodies of neurons located in the *sacral segments* of the spinal cord

iii. *Terminal ganglia*:

- are ganglia that lie near or within the target organ that it innervates
- postganglionic parasympathetic fibers synapse in terminal ganglia

C. Autonomic Plexuses

- associated with the autonomic nervous system are branching network of nerves that are comprised of branches of preganglionic and postganglionic nerve fibers

III. Functional Organization of the Autonomic Nervous System

A. Sympathetic System

I. Distribution of Preganglionic Neurons (Figure 21.1):

- cell bodies of preganglionic neurons of the sympathetic division of the autonomic nervous system are located in the *intermediolateral cell column* of the *lateral gray horns* of T1 to T12 segments and L1 to L2 or L3 segments of the spinal cord
- sympathetic preganglionic fibers are referred to as the *thoracolumbar outflow* (Figure 21.2)
- preganglionic fibers are myelinated and leave the spinal cord via the ventral root of a spinal nerve, travel for a short distance within the spinal nerve and leave the spinal nerve to extend to a corresponding sympathetic ganglion via a short pathway called a *white communicating ramus*. White communicating rami are white because preganglionic fibers are myelinated.
- sympathetic preganglionic fibers synapse with many postganglionic neurons that innervate several visceral effectors, therefore sympathetic stimulation is widespread throughout the body

II. Distribution of Postganglionic Neurons (Figure 21.1):

1. Preganglionic axons that enter the paravertebral sympathetic ganglion through the white ramus terminate on its target organ in one of the following pathways:

a. some preganglionic sympathetic fibers synapse in the ganglion of the sympathetic trunk. Postganglionic fibers from the sympathetic ganglion exit the ganglion to enter T1-L2 spinal nerves via a short pathway called the *gray communicating ramus*. Gray communicating rami are gray since they contain unmyelinated fibers. Most of the structures of the body wall, such as the sweat glands, arrector pili muscle and blood vessels of the skin and skeletal muscles receive their innervation by this pathway.

b. some preganglionic fibers ascend or descend within the sympathetic trunk before synapsing in another sympathetic ganglion thereby allowing sympathetic outputs to supply structures that lie superiorly or inferiorly, such as the structures of the head and pelvis

c. some preganglionic fibers pass through the sympathetic trunks and exit the sympathetic trunk without synapsing to form the *splanchnic nerves*. Splanchnic nerves terminate in *prevertebral ganglia*. Postganglionic fibers innervate abdominal and pelvic viscera by this pathway (Figure 21.2).

2. Sympathetic preganglionic fibers also innervate the *adrenal medulla* which are modified postganglionic sympathetic neurons that secrete the hormones norepinephrine and epinephrine

B. Parasympathetic System

I. Distribution of Preganglionic Neurons:

• cell bodies of the preganglionic neurons of the parasympathetic division of the autonomic division are located in the *cranial nerve nuclei* of the midbrain, pons and medulla oblongata (associated with the oculomotor, facial, glossopharyngeal and vagus nerves) and the *lateral gray horns* of the second through the fourth sacral segments of the spinal cord
• preganglionic parasympathetic fibers are referred to as the *craniosacral outflow* (Figure 21.3). Fibers that arise from the *cranial nerve nuclei* are called the *cranial outflow* and fibers that arise from the *sacral segments* of the spinal cord are called the *sacral outflow*
• parasympathetic preganglionic fibers synapse with fewer postganglionic neurons, there is less divergence and parasympathetic effects tend to be localized

a. *Cranial outflow*

The cranial parasympathetic outflow includes five cranial nerve autonomic nuclei. Review the locations and details of cranial nerve nuclei and nerves

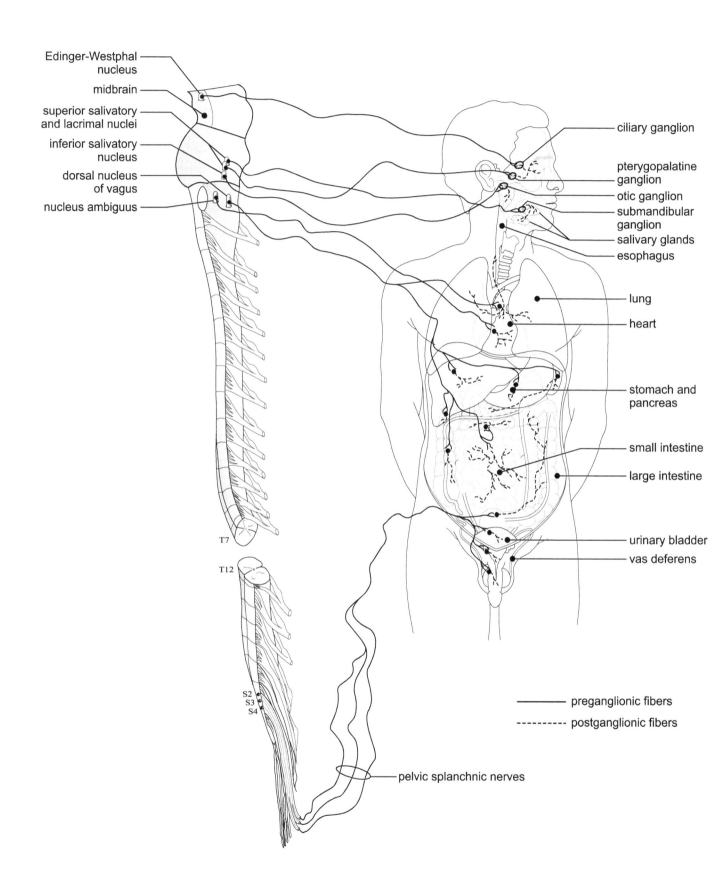

Figure 21.3   Parasympathetic Nervous System

in Chapter 8

Preganglionic *cranial nerve autonomic nuclei* (Figure 8.1) located in the brainstem are as follows:

    i.   *Edinger-Westphal nucleus*: preganglionic fibers leave the midbrain through the oculomotor nerve

    ii.   *superior salivatory nucleus* and *lacrimal nucleus*: preganglionic fibers leave the pons through the facial nerve

    iii.   *inferior salivatory nucleus*: preganglionic fibers leave the medulla through the glossopharyngeal nerve

    iv.   *dorsal nucleus of the vagus*: preganglionic fibers leave the medulla through the vagus nerve

    v.   *nucleus ambiguus*: preganglionic fibers leave the medulla through the vagus nerve

b. *Sacral outflow* (Figure 21.3)

- preganglionic parasympathetic fibers leave the spinal cord through the ventral roots of S2-S4 nerves and emerge collectively as the *pelvic splanchnic nerves*

II.   Distribution of Postganglionic Neurons:

a. *Cranial Parasympathetic System* (Figure 21.3)

    i.   preganglionic parasympathetic fibers leave the oculomotor nerve, synapse in the *ciliary ganglion* and supply the sphincter pupillae and ciliary muscle and functions in the accommodation reflex

    ii.   preganglionic parasympathetic fibers leave the facial nerve, synapse in the *submandibular ganglion* and *pterygopalatine ganglion* to supply the submandibular and sublingual salivary glands and the lacrimal gland

    iii.   preganglionic parasympathetic fibers leave the glossopharyngeal nerve, synapse in the *otic ganglion* and supply the parotid salivary gland

    iv.   preganglionic parasympathetic fibers leave the vagus nerve, synapse in the *terminal ganglia* within the wall of the thoracic and abdominal viscera to supply the organs of the thoracic and abdominal cavities (Figure 8.17)

b. *Sacral Parasympathetic System*

- preganglionic parasympathetic fibers leave the sacral splanchnic nerves, synapse in the *terminal ganglia* within the wall of the abdominal (descending colon and rectum) and pelvic viscera to supply smooth muscle and glands of the abdominal and pelvic viscera

IV. Functions of the Sympathetic and Parasympathetic System

1. The *sympathetic system* responds in times of stress and the generalized effects
    of sympathetic stimulation in a fight or flight response are:
    *bronchodilation, increase in heart rate, increase in blood flow to skeletal muscles,
    dilation of the pupils, decrease motility and blood flow of the gastrointestinal tract.*

2. The *parasympathetic system* responds during a restful state and the generalized
    effects of parasympathetic stimulation are:
    *decrease in heart rate, constriction of the pupils, increase in secretion and peristalsis
    of the gastrointestinal tract, contraction of the urinary bladder*

V. Neurotransmitters of the Autonomic Nervous System

a. *Cholinergic neurons* are
    -   all parasympathetic and sympathetic preganglionic axons
    -   all parasympathetic postganglionic neurons
    -   postganglionic sympathetic axons that supply sweat glands and arrector pili muscles

    Cholinergic neurons release acetylcholine that bind with *nicotinic receptors* or
    muscarinic receptors on the postsynaptic neuron leading to excitation or inhibition
    of the autonomic response

b. *Adrenergic neurons* are:
    -   sympathetic postganglionic neurons

    Adrenergic neurons release norepinephrine that bind to *alpha receptors* or *beta
    receptors* on the postsynaptic neuron to bring about excitation or inhibition of the
    autonomic response

c. *Interneurons*
    -   interneurons secrete *dopamine* and *neuromodulators* that enhance or inhibit the
        effect of acetylcholine or norepinephrine

Clinical Notes:

Several drugs either inhibit or stimulate the action of cholinergic or adrenergic
neurons, for example, a drug that can block *muscarinic receptors* in the stomach
is used to decrease acid secretion in patients suffering from peptic ulcer

VI. Enteric Nervous System

The Enteric Nervous System consists of plexus of cells and nerves forming an ***intrinsic network*** within the wall of the gastrointestinal tract.

  i.   the enteric nervous system consists of a plexus of unipolar, bipolar and multipolar neurons, neuroglial cells, preganglionic parasympathetic axons and postganglionic sympathetic axons

  ii.   plexuses in the wall of the gastrointestinal tract are located in two layers. The ***meissner's (submucosal) plexus*** lies in the submucosa and the ***myenteric (Auerbach's) plexus*** lies between the circular and longitudinal smooth muscle layers.

  iii.   the enteric system contain many cholinergic preganglionic fibers and cholinergic postganglionic parasympathetic neurons. All noradrenergic fibers are axons of sympathetic postganglionic neurons

  iv.   neurons of the meissner's plexus allows for movement of water and ions across the intestinal epithelium, neurons of the myenteric plexus controls motility of the gastrointestinal tract.

  v.   activity of the gut is also modulated by the sympathetic and parasympathetic divisions of the autonomic nervous system.

Clinical Notes:

Hirschsprung's disease is a congenital condition in which there is absence of the myenteric plexus in the distal part of the colon. In this condition there is hypertrophy and dilation of the colon, peristalsis is absent and the passage of feces is affected

VII. Central Nervous System Control of the Autonomic Nervous System

1. The ***hypothalamus*** is the main center for regulation of autonomic function in the central nervous system.
     i.   descending pathways from the hypothalamus synapse in autonomic cranial nerve nuclei of the brainstem and autonomic nuclei of the spinal cord. Ascending pathways from the spinal cord and brainstem relay information of visceral origin
     ii.   the *anterior portion* of the hypothalamus control parasympathetic functions. Stimulation of this region results in various parasympathetic responses.
     iii.   the *posterior portion* of the hypothalamus control sympathetic functions. Stimulation of this region results in various sympathetic responses
2. The ***prefrontal cortex*** is the main cortical area that influences autonomic response during emotional stress, via the structures of the limbic system that is brought about through its connections to the hypothalamus.
3. Cortical influence on visceral function can be achieved by biofeedback, for example, biofeedback training is used to manage stress or to control migraines

VIII. Distribution of General Visceral Afferent fibers of the Autonomic Nervous System

I. *Functional Considerations*

Afferents from the thoracic and abdominal viscera travel with autonomic pathways to relay to the central nervous system.   Visceral afferents include:

  a. afferents from viscera that are involved in reflexes that control important functions, such as circulation, respiration, digestion and micturition. *Visceral reflexes* are conveyed via parasympathetic fibers that travel with the *glossopharyngeal*, *vagus* and *pelvic splanchnic nerves*. Each ***autonomic visceral reflex*** arc consists of a *receptor*, a *sensory neuron*, *integrating center* in the central nervous system, two *autonomic motor neurons* and *visceral effector* (smooth muscle, cardiac muscle or glands)
  b. afferents from the viscera convey ***pain***, for example, constriction of a portion of the viscera can be perceived as cramping pain. Visceral pain from the thoracic and abdominal organs is conveyed by the ***sympathetic system*** via ***splanchnic nerves***

II. *Anatomic Pathways*

A. Visceral Afferents

Refer to Chapter 8 for details on the two pathways described below

  i. general visceral afferent fibers from ***baroreceptors*** (carotid sinus, aortic sinus) and ***chemoreceptors*** (carotid body, aortic body) are conveyed via the ***glossopharyngeal nerve*** and the ***vagus nerve*** (Figures 8.15, 8.16) for reflex control of respiration and blood pressure
  ii. general visceral afferent fibers are conveyed from the laryngeal mucosa, trachea and the thoracoabdominal viscera via the ***vagus nerve*** for subconscious reflex adjustment of the activity of regional viscera. Conscious influence of autonomic functions are possible through various connections between the cortex, hypothalamus and autonomic nuclei
  iii. general visceral afferent fibers conveyed from the descending colon, rectum and urinary bladder via the ***pelvic splanchnic nerves*** stimulate emptying of contents of the colon and the urinary bladder

B. Visceral Pain

Refer to Chapter 7 for details on the types of pain. Activation of nociceptors in internal organs as a result of tissue damage due to inadequate blood flow or muscle spasms is perceived as ***visceral pain***. Types of visceral pain are:

a. ***Pure visceral pain*** is described as pain that is felt deep to the skin, in the region of the affected viscera, for example, distension of the bile duct from a gallstone.

b. ***Referred pain*** is pain that arises from the viscera but is felt at a site on the surface of the body, different from its site of origin.

Two examples are:

i. impulses from an inflamed appendix is relayed through sympathetic fibers that terminate in T10 segment of the spinal cord; this pain is referred to an area around the umbilicus. The area of the umbilicus and the appendix are both innervated by T10 segment of the spinal cord.

ii. pain originating from a heart attack is felt along the skin of the left shoulder, substernal area and the medial side of the left arm since both the heart and the areas of skin are supplied by T1-T5 segments of the spinal cord.

Clinical Notes:

Autonomic dysfunction can have widespread effects on major structures of the body and can result in life threatening situations. Two clinical examples are:

i. ***Horner's syndrome***
Interruption of sympathetic innervation to the head and neck results in constriction of the pupil, drooping of the eyelid (ptosis) and loss of sweating

ii. ***Raynaud's disease*** is a disorder that is often triggered by exposure to cold resulting in constriction of the peripheral arteries of the upper limbs. Vasoconstriction can result in discoloration and pain of the extremities.

Printed in the USA
CPSIA information can be obtained
at www.ICGtesting.com
CBHW080034210724
11912CB00014B/948

9 781077 336001